LOSE
WEIGHT
4LIFE

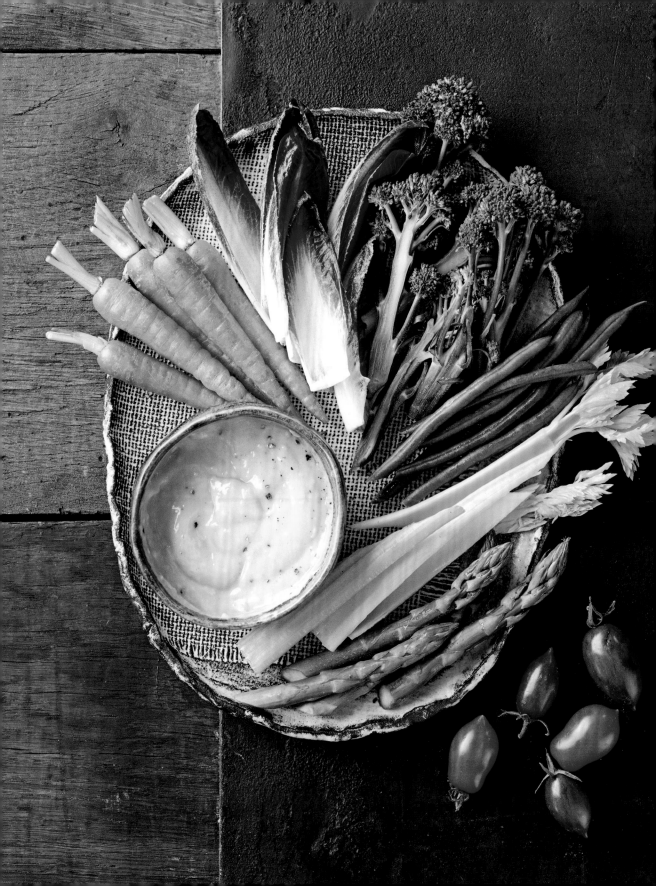

LOSE
WEIGHT
4LIFE

An Hachette UK Company
www.hachette.co.uk

First published in Great Britain in 2022 by Kyle Books,
an imprint of Octopus Publishing Group Limited
Carmelite House
50 Victoria Embankment
London EC4Y 0DZ

ISBN: 9781914239212

Publishing Director: Judith Hannam
Publisher: Joanna Copestick
Editor: Samhita Foria
Design: Paul Palmer-Edwards
Food styling: Lizzie Harris
Props styling: Faye Wears
Production: Lisa Pinnell

A Cataloguing in Publication record for this title is available
from the British Library.

Printed and bound in China

10 9 8 7 6 5 4 3 2 1

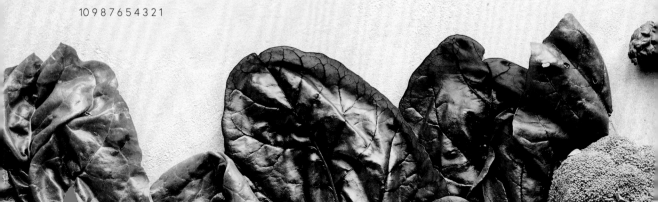

CONTENTS

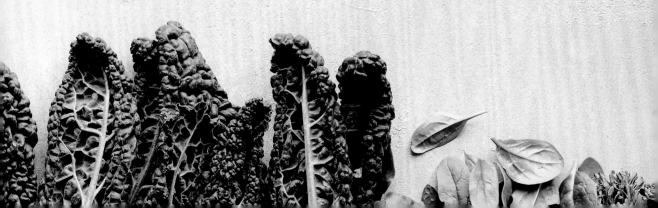

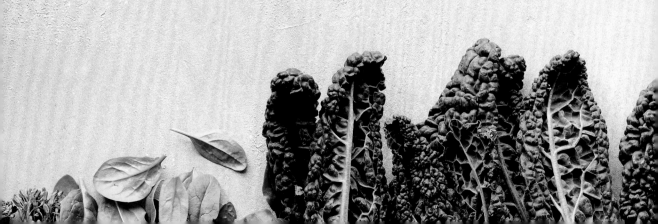

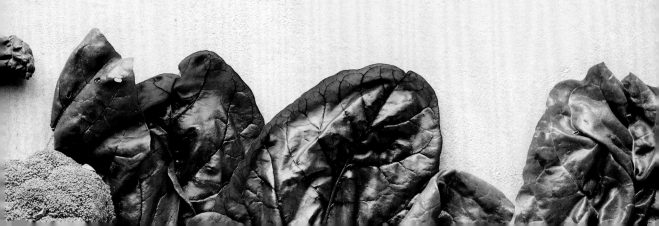

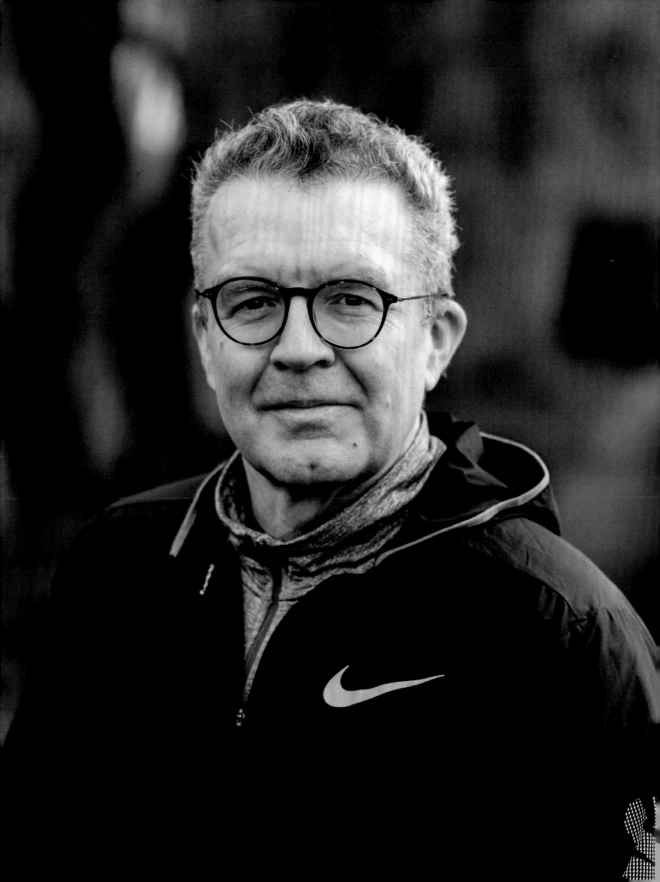

A reformed sugar addict

I'm Tom, and I'm a sugar addict.

Well, a reformed one these days, but at one point it was an addiction that nearly killed me.

My obsession with the sweet stuff – and with food in general, especially curries – earned me the nickname 'Tommy Two Dinners' as an MP and a type 2 diabetes diagnosis. To outsiders I may have appeared unconcerned about my weight but the truth was I felt overwhelmed by shame, embarrassment and fear.

The glimpse of a packet of chocolate biscuits on a supermarket shelf still makes me salivate. In fact, just thinking about them makes me euphoric. But ditching sugar completely has transformed my life. I've gone from being a morbidly obese dad weighing 22 stone (140kg), with zero stamina to play football with my kids, to one who is a healthy weight, completes 5k runs and can cycle for miles without gasping for breath.

What's more, I've reversed my type 2 diabetes. Before, things had got so bad I risked not having a future at all. Now I've got my future back, and can enjoy experiences that (at my heaviest) I never thought possible. Like the buzz from riding a bike – or just being able to get on one. Waking up in the morning with a clear head and plenty of energy is a reason to be thankful for the new me.

My transformation was down to a combination of healthy eating, a more positive mindset, getting motivated to change my habits and making movement part of my everyday routine. Walking is now a must for me, even if it means 5,000 steps instead of taking the car to the gym. There was never one single point of motivation, but my children were one of the most important factors. I didn't want to die – I wanted to live for them.

For a recent TV documentary, the producers asked me to jog around a racetrack wearing a vest weighing 20kg – or 50kg including the backpack and other accessories. The point of the exercise was that the kit represented the excess weight I had been carrying before downsizing. Wearing it made me realise the scale of the journey I had undertaken and how I never ever want to go back there again.

The aim of this book

It's important to make clear from the outset what this book ISN'T. First, it's neither a strict diet plan that involves you eating lots of weird stuff (although you will need to say goodbye to your sugar habit). Nor is it a sales pitch to get you to spend lots of money on products that don't work. And it's definitely not about quick fixes that won't last.

Opposite, clockwise from top left: On holiday in Majorca. A giant rugby top from my friend, Dave Anderson MP. Taking the wheel on a boating holiday. Tired at Manchester's snow dome.

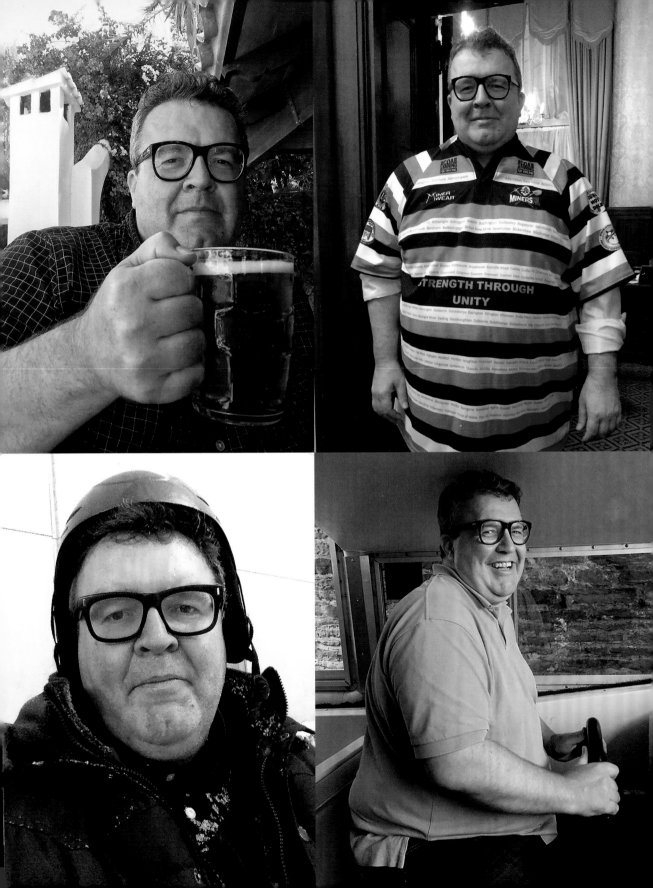

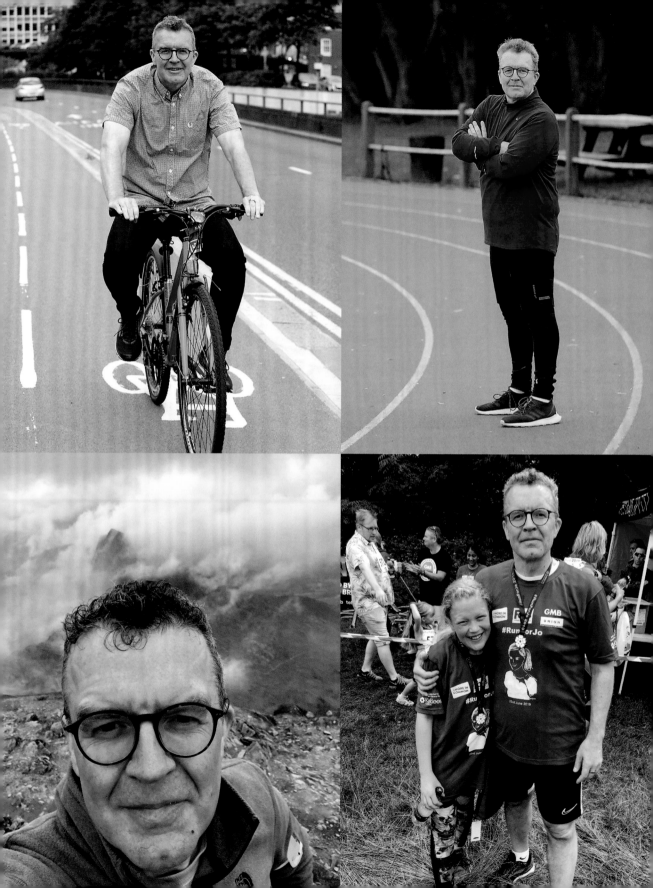

I've also done all I can to avoid sounding preachy. No one likes to be told off or lectured about their lifestyle when they feel bad enough about it already. Blame and criticism won't help – it makes the situation worse.

What *Lose Weight 4 Life* IS about is giving you a programme of helpful advice to assist you in losing weight long term. A handy blueprint for how you can change the habits of a lifetime. Throughout the book you'll find tips, recipes, easy-to-digest medical facts on what does and doesn't work (and why), plus bite-sized advice from the experts. I've also included simple food swaps that mean you don't need to give up what you like, you just need to switch to a healthier version that won't clog up your arteries.

For me, the road to shedding the excess pounds has been long and bumpy. So I've also shared personal (and sometimes cringeworthy) anecdotes from my own journey – and the journal I kept charting my progress – to help you realise you're not alone. My mother-in-law's favourite memory is of me with the fridge door open, eating half a block of cheese while talking on my mobile phone. A friend also witnessed me in a restaurant leaning over to the next table, picking up and demolishing a half-eaten slice of rainbow cake.

Opposite, clockwise from top left: Opening a new cycle lane in Birmingham. Filming for ITV. With my daughter Saoirse at the run for Jo Cox. At the summit of Snowdon.

On both occasions, I was totally unaware of what I was doing. It was behaviour created by my compulsive desire for food. Whether I was hungry or not, sating the craving dominated my life, sucked up time and wasted mental energy.

Failure doesn't mean the game's over

Even if you've failed to change your eating behaviour at every previous attempt, then do read on. In fact, that's even more reason to carry on reading. The reference to '4 life' is deliberate – the tips, targets and behaviour changes outlined in this book are for ever.

Losing 8 stone (50kg) taught me that it's not about the destination but the journey. Reaching a weight-loss goal or health target is very often the biggest challenge you will ever face. That inner voice deceives you, and it declares victory. The battle is over, it whispers. You've cracked it. Yet, the truth is that your biggest struggle has only just begun. How do you embed hard-fought habits and behaviours for life? How do you maintain emotional focus when you have setbacks? We all have them, and the temptation to slip back into your old life is never far away.

The pandemic lockdowns we have all endured in recent years have been disastrous for millions. The third national lockdown was nearly catastrophic for me. A new home, a new job and then a lockdown crushed all my hard-won habits and routines. Worst of all, my hastily assembled home office was just a few feet away from a fridge full of cheese. At one point, I was eating cheese like I used to scoff chocolate biscuits. I was slipping into unconscious, disordered eating again. My weight nudged up. I nearly dived deep into an ocean of denial like I had done for the previous thirty years when a diet inevitably failed.

Fortunately, this time around I understood what was going on. It took a bit of time, but I managed to reset my programme. I set new targets. I monitored my food and went back to collecting daily measurements. I discussed my new set of aims with friends, loved ones and work colleagues to remain accountable.

Thankfully, this has worked, and my weight is heading back in the right direction. I'm lifting weights back at the gym, I'm hitting my steps targets on most days and I feel in control.

If you find yourself falling back into old ways, then, as I have done, address it with a reset. There will always be curve balls that disrupt our lives. You can get back on track and be your best self with the help of my four mantras:

Motivation, **Movement**, **Measurement**, **Maintenance**.

My hope is that the insights, experience and advice I detail in this book will enable you to achieve and maintain your weight-loss goal. Whatever life throws at you.

Good luck! Now let's get started.

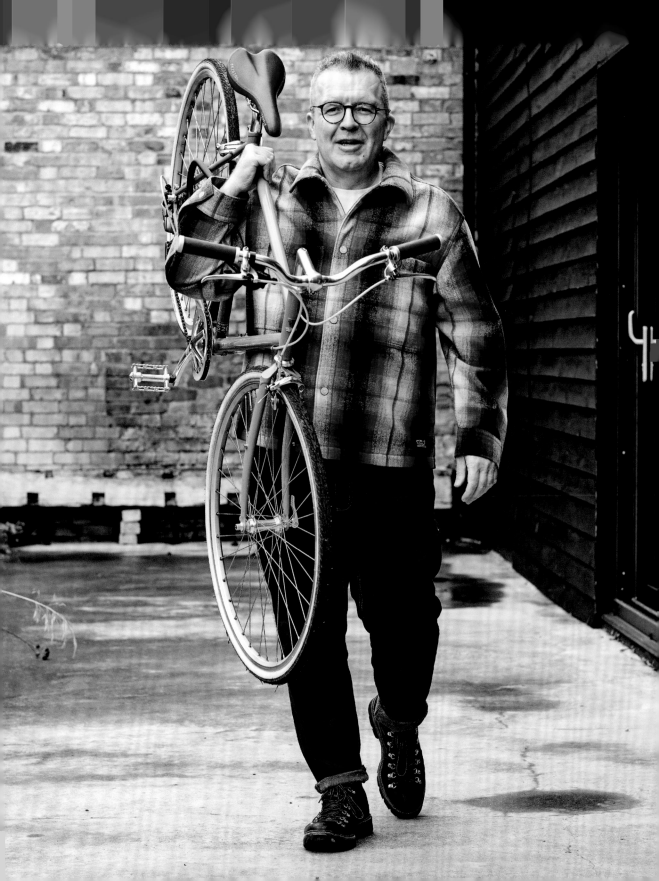

1 Motivation

Motivation is going to help you change your life. But it is a finite resource that should be deployed sparingly. Using your motivation to identify and destroy bad habits and to create new ones is worthwhile. Using willpower to resist temptation over the long term is a waste of your time and energy. You cannot achieve a permanent lifestyle change with willpower alone. Sooner or later you'll be giving in to 'yes' instead of saying 'no'. The sort of modifications you will have to make to transform yourself could last for decades. But they take time and dedication.

Self-control and willpower aren't enough

Finding the resolve to alter your eating habits is the first step on your weight-loss journey. You need to really *want* to do this. It's simple to say but not as easy to achieve. The second step is using your reserves of willpower to maintain these changes. Eventually, they will become habits, like brushing your teeth every day or changing your underwear.

Think about giving up two cans of fizzy drink a week at the age of 40. That's 280 calories or 78g of sugar you'd be cutting out. If you live until aged 80, you would prevent more than 160kg or 80 bags of refined sugar from going into your body.

Then imagine staring at a chilled can on a scorching summer day. There's the can in the fridge, droplets of ice-cold water forming around the tin, as on the adverts. Imagine having to stop yourself from flicking open the ring pull and guzzling down the fizzy liquid to quench your thirst.

Does just reading the last sentence bring back memories of doing this in childhood? It's powerful, right? You probably imagined the adverts as you read this paragraph, too.

Now think about having to stop yourself drinking the can in the fridge twice a week for 40 years.

You're being set up to fail.

The only way you can succeed is to use your motivation to reorganise your life in a way that means you are not tempted by this or any other calorific treat. That's why habits are so important.

It's also why, when you do fail, as you inevitably will at some point, you can't afford to lose motivation. It's motivation that is going to get you through the hours and days when you've fallen off the programme. And everyone, no matter how desperate they are to shed the weight, falls off the programme.

At the time of writing this chapter I'm on a reset myself. Lockdown three in the bleak UK winter months was a disaster for me. It disrupted my daily routines and habits to the point where my weight started to head in the wrong direction. The challenge for me, and for anyone trying to downsize, is that willpower may get you over the first hurdles, but it's not enough to carry you further.

It takes a 30-minute brisk walk to work off a 330ml can of fizzy drink.

Where there's a will, there's a way

Willpower is a finite resource. Think of it as a bank account. Where you invest your willpower is essential. Misuse it, and you will soon be in overdraft and back on the doughnuts. Instead of using it to resist eating particular foods, use it to work out how to avoid temptation. Your willpower should be used to deploy creative solutions to identified problems, no matter how tiny they seem. I ask my family to permanently hide crisps and eat them when I'm not around. In the end, they do this because they know I'm likely to eat their crisps if they leave them within eyesight! It sounds silly, but it works – most of the time.

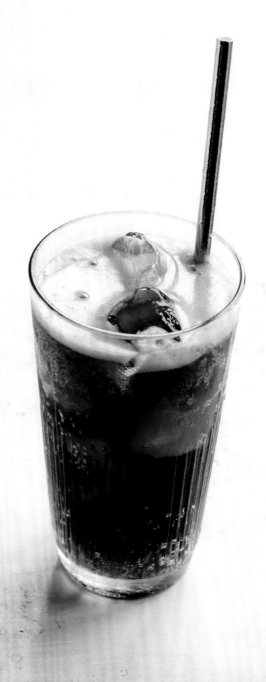

Eating a packet of crisps a day is the equivalent of drinking 5.5 litres of cooking oil a year.

Lack of determination was never an issue for me when it came to wanting to win elections and trounce the political opposition. Or when writing speeches. But finding the will to look after my health and eating less? Well, that's another matter, especially when temptation is all around.

For 30 years, I couldn't lose weight. Each time I tried I thought my self-control would kick in, only to end up deceived and despondent. What was missing was knowledge, time management and organisation. And knowing the difference between good habits and bad.

There are several factors at play in achieving a goal. Humans are guided by their emotions, biology and the mind, with external and internal influences pushing them in a specific direction. Mine pushed me in the direction of the nearest snack.

What's key is taking practical steps to keep you on track, such as identifying unhealthy habits, making time in your day to eat properly and adopting simple life hacks to retrain your mind.

Processed food – the ingredients test

Check the back of the packets of food in your fridge or cupboard. How many ingredients do they list on the label? If the answer is 'a lot' then it's likely to be processed. Salt, sugar and fat have all been added to make it more appealing, but that means more calories. And if there are five or more ingredients, then alarm bells should really start ringing, because what you're looking at is ultra-processed food, products that are packed with high-energy additives, preservatives and other baddies that provide almost zero nutrients. In his book *Metabolical*, Dr Robert Lustig reveals that 62% of food in US supermarkets is ultra-processed. And added sugar is the key component driving the risk of health problems such as type 2 diabetes, heart disease and cancer. The physician, who treats childhood diabetes, says 'Ultra-processed products are made to be hyper-palatable and attractive, with long shelf-life, and able to be consumed anywhere, any time. Their formulation, presentation and marketing often promote overconsumption.'

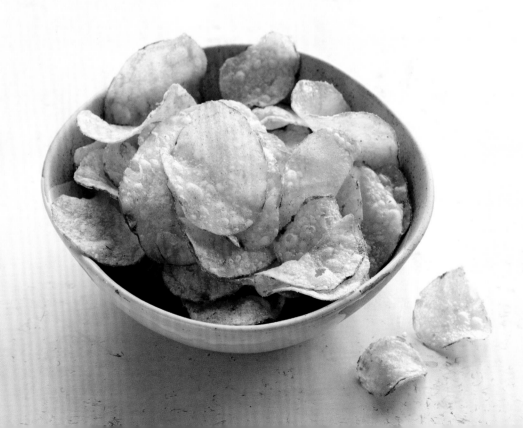

Recognising unhealthy habits

If you don't think deeply about your habits – I mean *really* analyse them – you will fail and you won't have the resilience to deal with the inevitable setbacks.

My food indiscretions were deeply ingrained. At social events, I'd move from table to table clearing whatever food was left on plates. I didn't even know I did this until told by colleagues and friends. Gregarious is my middle name, so I thought I was just being sociable and getting to talk to as many people as possible. The truth was it was a good excuse to hoover up extra (but empty) calories at the same time. So the first habit that had to go was grazing on fat-making food. That meant a kitchen 'detox': emptying my fridge, freezer and cupboards, even of things within the sell-by date.

The art of the kitchen 'detox'

Cancelling the carbs, saying 'no' to sugar and parting with processed junk. These were all on my list of habits that had to change. The first step was to clear out my cupboards. Nearly everything had to go, including half-eaten packets of breakfast cereal bought for the children and jams they'd barely used (but I did when desperate). I ended up filling two black bin-liners. This sounds drastic/expensive and of course I was quivering with low-level angst at throwing out 'good' food that I'd paid for. The clear-out, though, cut my chances of reverting to unhealthy habits, such as scoring a sneaky sugar fix. Even donating to the food bank was off limits in case I didn't get round to parting with my offerings. For the first time in years, my cupboards contained no unhealthy food, and I didn't look back.

What had to go
- all rice and pasta
- processed dry food, such as noodle pots
- oven chips
- ice cream
- ultra-processed foods, such as microwave meals
- hidden-sugar and/or high-carb items, for example, baked beans
- high-sugar foods, including jam, marmalade, breakfast cereal
- bread
- high-sugar content alcohol, such as beer

What I swapped them for
- meat
- fish
- eggs
- vegetables, such as cauliflower 'rice'
- butter and lots of olive oil
- low-sugar alcohol, such as vodka

Tips for a kitchen clear-out

- Empty out ALL your cupboards
- Arrange the contents on newspaper on the floor
- Put all the items that have to go into bin bags

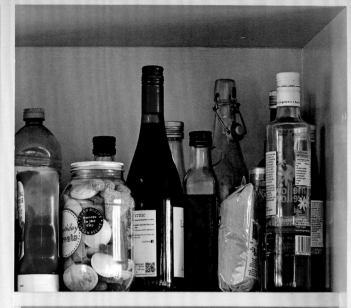

- Take the bags STRAIGHT to the bin store (and don't return… or the food will creep back into your cupboards)
- Do the same with your fridge and freezer
- Do a shop the same day to restock with healthy food

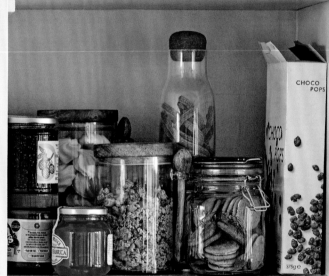

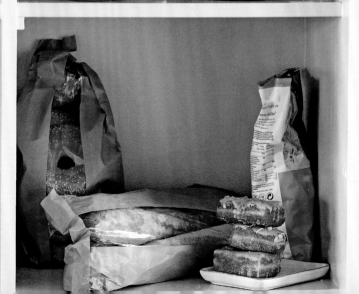

Adapting your diet

On good days, post clear-out, I was eating meat and five different veg. It was the type of food my grandparents would have eaten: fresh, simple and without additives. Of course, they may also have eaten boiled sweets, but overall their refined sugar intake would have been much lower than the amount most of us consume today.

Some of my new-look store cupboard essentials were bags of pecans and walnuts. Nuts are high in fat, which at first made me freak out – I was convinced I'd add even more weight to my super-sized body. The message here is that it takes time to adapt. The food you now need to eat will seem alien. Habits are hard to break, but with the right motivation, it can be done and you will be better for making the change. Today, nuts are one of my favourite snacks. I've been converted.

Bad
Basmati rice

Better
Frozen cauliflower rice

Best
Home-cooked cauliflower rice with added vegetables

Food Swaps

Swap pepperoni cheese pizza for tomato pizza with diced chicken and mushrooms

Swap potato chips for halloumi chips

Swap curry with biryani rice for curry with cauliflower rice

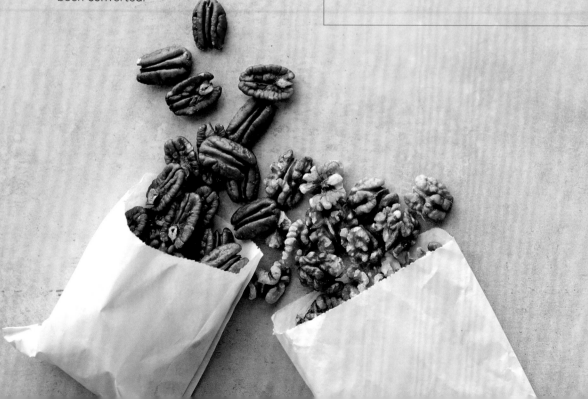

100g of jelly sweets
= approx. 50g of sugar
or the equivalent of
1 teaspoon per sweet.

Finding and (taking) the time to be healthy

The downside of ditching a junk-food diet is the extra time spent preparing food from scratch. A takeaway or microwaved evening meal takes minutes to order or heat up, whereas a home-cooked dinner of meat or fish takes considerably longer. The same is true for breakfast. I switched from a 2-minute high-sugar cereal fix to spending 20 minutes preparing a cooked plate of food, albeit one that wouldn't leave me with cravings or result in a mid-morning slump (see the chapter on Diets, page 42). Fresh food also deteriorates faster than products packed with chemical preservatives, so I had to be much more organised with my shopping and had to learn to keep the fridge stocked.

At first, I felt the extra minutes spent cooking and buying food was time stolen from me. Then something happened. My mindset gradually shifted from resentment to enjoyment. The task of preparing food became an opportunity to allow my thoughts to roam freely while I peeled and chopped. There are countless other upsides to packing in the bad stuff and switching to nutritious meals, not least the fact that you know what went into them. Food also tastes so much better when you make it yourself, plus doing so can give you deep sense of satisfaction.

What about the cost? There's a perception that fresh ingredients cost more than buying ready-prepared meals. The reality is I found myself spending less money because real home-cooked food is cheaper than home-delivered takeaways. The raw ingredients might be cheap for the takeaway firms but there's a massive mark-up on the end product. How often have you got change out of £60 after ordering a dinner delivery for a family of four? Not me. I found I could feed my kids for an entire weekend, including providing a full Sunday lunch, if I bought the ingredients and cooked the meals myself from scratch.

Getting family, friends and colleagues on board
– as well as yourself!

When my downsizing journey began, I was living alone in London most of the time, which made life easier. There were no negotiations to be had about cupboard contents or tense situations involving others eating forbidden foods in front of me. I controlled what foods were allowed through the front door.

This won't be the case for everyone reading this book. If you share accommodation, asking flat/housemates to hide bad foods away so they're not in your eyeline can be a solution. I lived with someone who used to conceal chocolate and sweets in the bottom of a tower of pans to stop me scoffing the lot. Such ruses aren't practical, though, if you have children in the house, nor is banning them from buying sweets or crisps.

Eating my kids' sweets was always a problem for me. I'm a sugar addict, right? I remember the night before one Easter Sunday when I thought I could just eat one (tiny) piece of egg. An hour later, I was sat in the living room surrounded by empty boxes and foil wrappers feeling utter shame.

My anxiety was lessened when I managed to communicate honestly with my family. If you can share your vulnerability with the people that matter, your life will be a lot easier. Discuss why you can no longer eat bad food, explain how serious you are about losing weight, and your fears about being overweight and unhealthy, which in my case included the conviction that I would die.

Luckily, they wanted me to succeed, but there had to be a conversation first about why I needed to restrict my diet. And that meant removing all the tempting stuff because my cravings were so great it couldn't be within my reach. The first weekend the kids came to visit my new eating regime was a bit weird for them. We went to a well-known fast-food chicken chain where I had a couple of plain chicken fillets. They also like burger joints and I don't want to impose my eating restrictions on them. The compromise that has worked for me (and is available in most high-street burger chains) is ordering a cheeseburger in a lettuce wrap (without the bun) and a bottle of water.

Communication is also necessary with colleagues. The tradition in many offices is to 'treat' everyone on your birthday by buying cakes. Or it was where I worked. To turn down a colleague's obesogenic 'gifts' or tell everyone they'd be no calorie-laden celebration of your birthday can seem rude or ungrateful. So, my strategy was to explain upfront I was trying to go sugar-free. And I'd suggest we avoid giving each other sweet temptations.

> The only person who knows how much you're eating is you.

Arranging your working day to fit in exercise does require negotiation. I had to clear my diary to make time for steps in the park. But they got more productive time out of me because I was more laid-back as a colleague.

With weight loss, there's another key person who you need to get real with, as I discovered from the outset. That person is you. It's all very well to reveal your mission to those around you and ask them for support. But the only person who really knows what and how much you're eating is you. Before I embarked on my downsizing programme, I was the master of self-deceit. I'd go to the tearoom in the House of Commons, eat a bacon butty and drink a mug of tea, then return 20 minutes later and do the same again. All the while telling myself the first time didn't really happen – because if you don't count the calories they don't really exist. Right?

Except that even if you succeed in cheating your mind, you won't deceive your body. So quit the fibs and the excuses. Be honest with *yourself* from the outset and take responsibility.

I had to identify the foods that created the dreaded moments of weakness. Ice cream is kryptonite for me – it only takes a spoonful and I'm off. It's always one spoonful at a time, eaten on multiple returns to the freezer. Before I'm aware of it, the whole tub is gone. In the end I knew I had just to stop eating ice cream altogether. It's no loss, but it requires clarity of thought to work out the patterns of eating and where my weaknesses lie.

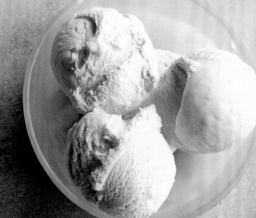

Mindset

Ditching the pounds is hard, as I know all too well. The road to shedding excess weight is a long one, with many setbacks on the way. You need to be mentally prepared for this and able to accept that nothing will happen overnight. But this isn't a reason to give up. If you make the effort to change the habits and behaviours you've formed over decades, probably as far back as childhood, anything is achievable. What's needed to make it happen is a *change of mindset*.

Motivation is the pathway to altering habits and behaviours. But you also need the self-belief and positive attitude to keep going on your journey. This is a major influencer of motivation. Understanding the relationship between your brain and food/eating is also an important part of this. This knowledge enables you to identify (and overcome) negative patterns and behaviours.

There are two types of mindset. The first is 'fixed' – this is the negative belief that your abilities and traits can't be changed. Then there's the positive 'growth' way of thinking, that you can develop yourself over time with effort and persistence. I'm not suggesting this means you're going to transform into an Olympic athlete.

What I am saying is that you can become a healthier and fitter person with the right approach. As Stanford University psychologist Carol Dweck has detailed, with a growth mindset you believe that your basic abilities can be developed, so you are more likely to learn more skills, and more quickly, but with a fixed mindset you are less likely to take on new challenges.

Make small changes (they will lead to big changes)

'Lose weight' will be top of the wishlist of anyone reading this book. Just those words are daunting. And they're probably not associated with good feelings.

A technique developed by behaviour scientist B J Fogg – who has spent more than 20 years researching human behaviour at Stanford University – is to lower the bar. As he explains in his book *Tiny Habits*, small changes accumulate over time to yield big results.

The trick is to make the tasks so small that they're easily accomplished. It's not a new technique but one that few of us practise properly – we're all guilty, for example, of leaving deadlines until the last minute so that they become worse, leaving us feeling sick with panic at the task ahead.

The trick is to make the tasks small enough that they are easily accomplished.

If you apply it to downsizing, you're more likely to feel positive and inclined to repeat the task. For example:

- Try parking in the spot furthest away from the supermarket entrance the next time you shop. You'll walk more and burn more calories.

- Or try to do a walk at lunchtime at least one day a week.

Always follow up these small changes by praising yourself. On page 36, I discuss how to create a reward system.

Small changes done repeatedly become routines that in turn become bigger habits. In his book *Atomic Habits*, James Clear talks about habit 'stacking', a process where you create a rule and then add to it. For example, if you do one press-up a day this leads to two, then three a day. And in my case 25, which over a year adds up to more than 1,000 (or about 3,000 calories).

Other 'small' habits I formed included taking regular measurements. I would make this happen by standing on the weighing scales while I put the kettle on to make a cup of coffee. Then I'd record my weight in the MyFitnessPal app on my phone. Part of the 'rule' was to high-five myself mentally if my weight hadn't increased.

Another challenge I set myself was to walk up every set of steps I came to. As well as the steps to my flat, this included the occasional stair at work. Then fate intervened: I was told by officials that I needed to move office – and urgently. So I found myself in a new office that could only be accessed by climbing 66 steps. At the first attempt I could barely breathe and my throat felt like it was on fire. And that was after just reaching the middle landing. By the time I stood down from Parliament just over two years later, I was *running* up and down the stairs.

At first it was tough, unnatural – even uncomfortable – to make this change. But eventually it became unnatural to take the lift. A small habit had turned into a bigger one and helped transform me. And it goes without saying I was so much fitter as a result.

Positive affirmation: how to ditch your inner critic

You are the only person judging yourself. People may be dismissive and make unkind comments or they may try to help with encouragement, but they're not the ones facing the task of a radical life edit. The only person you really need to do battle with on your journey is your own inner voice.

It can be a harsh critic.

We all beat ourselves up from time to time, some more than others. But when this becomes self-destructive it's time to bring some positive affirmation into your life. The trick is to 'reverse' the conversation by changing negative and self-sabotaging thoughts into positive ones. Mindfulness can help quiet your inner voice. Other techniques to change your behaviour include neuro-linguistic programming and cognitive behavioural therapy (CBT).

CBT was a huge deal for me in reaching my downsizing goal. Take food preparation. Instead of telling myself this was a chore, I celebrated the fact it gifted me time to think as I cooked. Another benefit was the cost-saving of eating real food, not takeaways.

The same applied to my partying ways. For years, me getting in before midnight would have been as rare as a sighting of Santa in summertime. Now, my aim was always to be in by a reasonable time. The natural response would have been for me to think I was missing out, that 'There's a party going on and I'm not there.' I turned this thought around by focusing on how lucky I was to get a decent night's sleep and how good I'd feel the next morning. In fact, getting a good night's sleep plays an important part in weight loss, one that I explain in more detail on page 130.

I've touched on habits, including identity being the most important level of change, according to James Clear's theory. In my mind, I was the fat guy. So who did I need to become? The answer was the person who committed to walking 10,000 steps a day. So I became that person. I committed to it by organising my time. I didn't start at that level (my target was 5,000), but by the end I was the guy for whom it was normal to take a walk after lunch. The guy who left their flat 20 minutes early to walk to the office. And the guy who had a proper night's sleep.

Change is possible with the right outlook.

Of course, your inner voice isn't going to give up without a fight. It will struggle, resist and rebel by planting the seeds of doubt. I had the weakest will when it came to resisting foods that made me fat and was on a fast track to early death, but if you get your head in the right place, you will succeed. And feel so much better as a result.

Practising mindfulness

Mindfulness is all about focusing on the now, paying more attention to the present moment – to your thoughts and feelings, to the world around you – and according to the NHS it can improve your mental wellbeing. No one is too busy to stop and think. For years I deluded myself that I didn't have the time to change my daily schedule. I was a busy politician, right? Yet reorganising my diary around exercise meant less time chatting to the takeaway delivery driver and at the corner shop and more time to walk or cycle around Kennington Park in London having conversations with myself.

You notice the natural world more when you're alone and not with busy people – the sun on your skin, the red of a robin's breast and the smell of mown grass. My senses were awakened by being outdoors doing my daily steps. And I began to derive pleasure from just being in the moment.

Despite growing up in Worcestershire in the shadow of the Wyre Forest, the only tree I could recognise was an oak. So I bought a book to learn more. Now, not only can I name many more trees than just oaks, I also have a deeper respect for the environment.

Professor Edith Hall's book, *Aristotle's Way*, details how we can all follow the example of the great Greek philosopher who was one of the first happiness gurus. His philosophy that living a meaningful life is the path to contentment (not wealth, possessions or fame) fits with concepts such as mindfulness. Hall has taken his ancient wisdom and repurposed it for modern living. Her tips are based around fully engaging with every encounter and decision, and the rich texture of life. Not by applying big rules and principles.

What is mindfulness?

Professor Mark Williams, former director of the Oxford Mindfulness Centre, defines mindfulness as knowing directly what is going on inside and outside ourselves, moment by moment. The technique has its roots in Buddhism and credits Jon Kabat-Zinn at the University of Massachusetts, among others, with kick-starting the Western movement, initially developed for stress-reduction and to treat the chronically ill. To get you started, here are three simple exercises:

- Breathe and smile – facial muscles will trigger the release of endorphins.

- Sit for 5 minutes – take this time to pay attention to sensations in your body.

- Inhale deeply, say 'let' to yourself. Then exhale deeply and say 'go'. Repeat this mantra until you feel relaxed.

Too many of us associate sugar with reward. It makes us feel good – at least in the short term.

Chewing it over: applying mindfulness to eating

As well as being more 'present' during my exercise sessions outdoors, I also became more fully aware, respectful and appreciative of the food on my plate, from the taste to the texture. That meant chewing it more and realising how lucky I was to have a freshly prepared meal. Previously, I wasn't really conscious of what went in my mouth, or why or how much. All I knew was that my brain was telling me I needed seconds and thirds. Or more.

Sugary sweets were banned on the diet plan I adopted, but I was allowed a small amount of dark chocolate. At first, the experience was like putting grit in my mouth because my brain was hardwired to expect the explosive hit that came from high-sugar treats. Now, thanks to mindful eating, the taste sensation from high (80%) cocoa solids chocolate is a million times more enjoyable than a sugar- and saturated-fat-laden bar of standard milk chocolate.

Combating cravings

The intense desire for certain foods – especially when you've given them up – can seem uncontrollable at times. This extreme response is 'learned' by our brains because we associate sugar with reward. It makes us feel good – at least in the short term. That's because eating the sweet stuff triggers levels of the brain chemical dopamine (see box opposite) to soar.

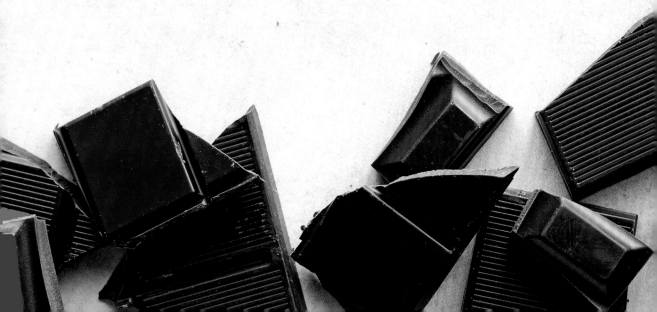

I craved many foods, but milk chocolate was the absolute killer for me. Just looking at an Easter egg used to make me drool. Then, when you unwrap the chocolate, there is the smell – another powerful trigger. With high-sugar milk chocolate, there is also a pleasant texture in the mouth as it melts on the palate. For me, by this point, moderation does not exist. As I type this paragraph, I still feel the shame of scoffing all my children's chocolate eggs on the night before Easter Sunday. Combating deeply held physical and psychological relationships with a particular food is tough, but you can do it.

For the ITV documentary *Giving Up Sugar: For Good?* I tasted sugar for the first time in three years since quitting. During filming, the crew recorded me eating chunks of milk chocolate, and by the end of the day I was getting sugar cravings. My brain was buzzing and I felt like I was on a drug. Which some experts will tell you is exactly what sugar is.

The science of chewing food

Digestion begins in the mouth. The more you munch on what's in your mouth, the smaller the pieces of food and the easier they are to break down. Taking time to chew properly also mixes what you're eating with saliva. A special enzyme in saliva helps to break down carbohydrates (starches) into sugars, which are easier for your body to absorb. And another enzyme is responsible for breaking down fats. There's some evidence that a slower eating pace may help weight loss. A study published in the *Journal of Consulting and Clinical Psychology* in 2019 found a programme combining mindfulness and prolonged chewing led to reductions in Body Mass Index (BMI).

So here are a few tips on how to slacken the pace at the dinner table:

• Put your cutlery down between bites.

• Sip on water.

• Talk to your fellow diners more.

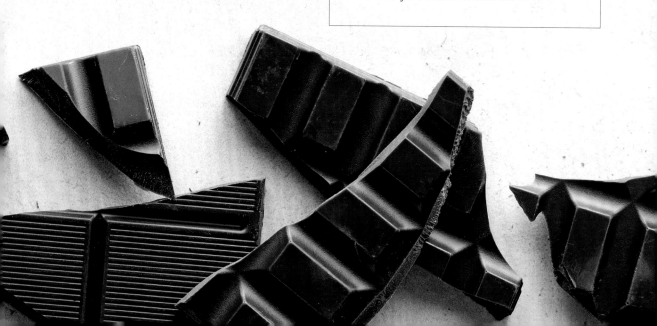

How to make bulletproof coffee

- Brew one cup (225–350ml) of coffee using 2½ heaped tablespoons of ground coffee beans. Use a cafétiere to preserve beneficial coffee oils that paper filters keep out.

- Add 1–2 tablespoons of MCT oil. Start with 1 teaspoon per cup and work your way up to 1–2 tablespoons over several days.

- Add 1–2 teaspoons of grass-fed, unsalted butter or grass-fed ghee.

- Mix it all in a blender for 20 seconds until it looks like a foamy latte.

For me, a bulletproof coffee seemed to level out the urge to reach for the nearest confectionery bar.

The high-calorie/low-carb drink made of butter, black coffee and MCT oil was pioneered by Dave Asprey, author of *The Bulletproof Diet*. MCT stands for medium-chain triglycerides, a type of fat which is thought to help support weight-loss. The aim is to make you feel satiated, alert and stop you hunting down the next sugar fix. Bulletproof coffee works with several types of diet, including ketogenic, paleo and low-carb, about which I provide more details in the next chapter. Whether it was a placebo effect or really helped, I don't know. But it's worth giving it a try to see if it works for you too.

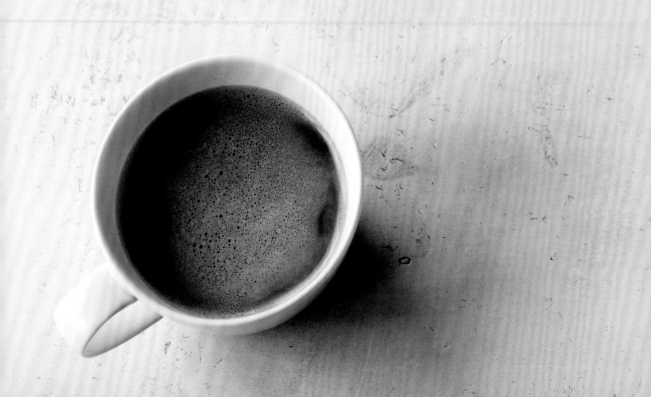

Owning setbacks

There will be times when your resolve weakens. The wine the host pours into your glass when you're busy chatting with friends around the dinner table. Or the bread roll the waiter puts on your plate at a wedding before you can say 'No thanks'.

Sometimes, you just can't help getting cornered. These are minor losses of focus in your weight-loss journey, but make sure you own them. My strategy was to log these and check the 'bad nutrient' tally. Then take the view that this was just a setback and tomorrow was another day to try again.

When you choose to overhaul your life, there will be many voices in your head vying for attention. Some positive, but often the negative ones are louder. Targets are milestones. You're on a never-ending journey and sometimes you will take steps forwards only then to end up going backwards. But remember, you're not a machine, you're a human being.

In moments of weakness or despair, it's helpful to focus on the experience of a role model who has overcome tough times to get fit. My personal hero – the guru in my head willing me on – is David Goggins, a former cockroach catcher who became a Navy SEAL. The American author of *Can't Hurt Me* once weighed 300lb (136kg) and endured numerous hardships, but he became a successful extreme athlete – he even ran a 100-mile race with a broken leg. His story is exceptional, and I'm not expecting you to join a crack military unit. But being inspired by someone like Goggins will spur you on after a blip in progress.

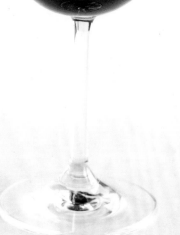

Bad
Binge eating

Better
Understanding why you respond to
a specific food

Best
Learning to control that response

Rewards and wins

Everyone needs praise, rewards and incentives, especially when trying to lose weight. Without them, you'll soon lose motivation.

You may already have heard of 'nudge' theory. This is based on the idea that subtle incentives – or 'nudges' – influence everyday behaviour. Fruit at eye level in supermarkets, smaller plate sizes and shopping vouchers for attending weight-loss programmes are among nudges drawn up by health experts to help curb the obesity crisis.

The uncomfortable truth, though, is that unhealthy food and drink are the rewards many of us turn to, especially after a hard week at work or when wanting to celebrate an important event. Or even after exercise – who hasn't bought a chocolate bar post-gym session as a treat for 'being good' and for burning all those calories (which you're now putting straight back on)?

When you're a food addict like me, anything related to eating sugar can lead to excess. Even now, I feel anxious being near cake because I know that I won't be able to stop after one bite.

So, the dilemma for downsizers is how do you incentivise yourself on your path to a healthier life? Thankfully, there are ways of 'high-fiving' yourself other than resorting to food. Everyone has their own definition of what counts as a treat. For some it could be buying yourself a new music album or booking yourself a massage.

How to high-five yourself at each milestone

A simple way to start is to record – or 'bank' – small wins in a diary or on your phone.

My own system was based around the reward of a bicycle. My main target was to lose 100lb (45.4kg). When I hit this goal after about nine months, I bought myself a new bicycle.

On the way to my main target, I had smaller milestones, each with a little prize for my old bike, such as new handlebar grips and a new bell. Also on the list of 'treats' was a basket that could be attached to the back of the bike. The significance of this was the bike was no longer just a tool for exercise, but also a useful means of doing the shopping and moving around the city.

Being able to buy clothes from somewhere other than outsize retailers was another reward. I was euphoric when, for the first time in 20 years, I was able to buy myself an off-the-peg suit and a pair of jeans at Marks & Spencer.

Shedding the pounds also meant I could finally fit into an XL Fred Perry polo shirt, eventually slimming down to fit into to a Large.

When more pounds had been shed, I was able to fit into a Medium. Even now I still swing between Medium and Large but the sense of satisfaction at having this dilemma is immense.

A picture of the new slimmed-down me at the Glastonbury music festival wearing my Fred Perry appeared in a Sunday newspaper next to an image of me at the same event several years earlier and many stones heavier. Despite this intrusion into my personal life, it was a picture to be proud of.

Of course, there will be days when you feel rubbish. This is inevitable. Don't beat yourself up or allow your inner critic to take over. You can still bank a mini win and say 'my old self couldn't have done that'. Even if it's just the fact that you've pledged to get back on the programme tomorrow.

Some examples of what I rewarded myself with when I hit weight-loss targets:

- A bell for my handlebars

- An iPhone grip for my bike

- A bike basket

- An XL Fred Perry Shirt

- When I lost 100lb, I treated myself to a new bike!

What is dopamine?

Professor Ciara McCabe, from Reading University, has been investigating the brain's reaction to the mere sight of food. The neuroscientist says that even advertising or packaging (or even the glimpse of a chocolate bar in my case) can trigger this response, which is linked to a chemical 'messenger' in the body called dopamine. This 'feel-good' neurohormone is released when your brain is expecting a reward. So when you associate an activity with pleasure, for example eating chocolate, dopamine levels rise in anticipation. We know this because tests show parts of the brain actually light up. Why is this bad? Too much dopamine is associated with poor impulse control, such as over-eating.

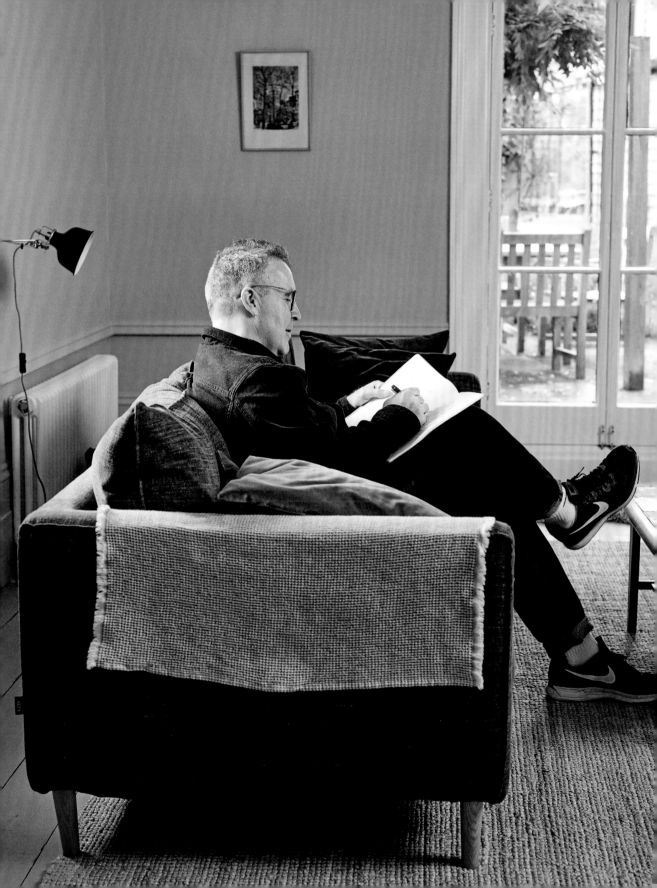

(December 28th)

The puppy is vaccinated now go on three 15 min day. I'm grateful for long walks for years +

(December 30th)

I'm grateful to my four Christmas beach walk by the sea and I bring about

---

Gratitude journal

To embed positive thoughts, try keeping a weekly gratitude journal to develop a more positive outlook.

Get yourself a notebook and write down:

- Pleasant surprises

- Good deeds you've done/benefited from

- Names of people you're grateful for in your life

- Experiences you've really enjoyed

- Challenging events you've overcome or that have increased your wisdom

Avoid becoming a hermit

Losing weight doesn't have to mean losing friends and missing out on fun. For the first month or so I turned down every invite, whether it was to the pub or a reception. Even speaking at fundraising dinners was off limits – I was on a journey, and I was desperately anxious to avoid being led astray from my weight-loss goal.

The reality, though, is that you can't cut yourself off from the world. It's not good for your mental health. And sooner or later you have to face temptation and learn how to deal with it. Inevitably, as I resumed a social life, I fell off the path. A curry with mates was often the flashpoint. The first couple of times I'd be disciplined, but then I'd find myself picking at a naan and half a poppadom. I would really punish myself afterwards and gloomily consider giving up the socialising. A more helpful response is to get the situation into perspective. This was just an aberration. Remember what I outlined about the power of motivation? Focus on changing your habits and mindset, not on beating yourself up mentally. Otherwise, your negative inner voice will take over and you'll become that 'bad' person. Perhaps next time opt for an extra portion of chicken tikka instead of the extra naan.

When you start, you'll be embarking on a solitary journey. It's all about you and the changes you are going to make. Some of your friends will come to represent temptation. Some of them will be jealous when you start to succeed. They may even try to sabotage what you are achieving without knowing it. I couldn't let that happen and, in the early weeks of my plan, I was often living hour by hour, fighting off cravings, organising and re-organising my routines to lay down habits, and thinking deeply about my goals. I was looking inwards and avoiding my usual social circles. It caused tension with some friends, but I told myself that my real friends would understand that I was improving my health.

However, you will eventually have to re-engage your social network. After about a month I would put occasional social events in my diary but continue to avoid all spontaneous activities, such as after-work drinks or last-minute lunch invitations. Even now, I still try to do that. It means that when you do have a night out, you appreciate the occasion.

IN SUMMARY

- Willpower alone won't get you through – recognise and deal with unhealthy habits, and control your response to temptation by learning about your relationship with food.

- Day one should focus on clearing out your kitchen cabinets, placing all 'toxic' food in a bin bag and then restocking with healthy food the same day. Remember, ultra-processed food has five or more ingredients and is especially high in salt and sugar.

- Communicate honestly with friends and family – and yourself – about your mission to lose weight and how you plan to achieve this goal.

- Adopt a positive mindset by believing you can develop yourself over time, ditch the inner critic, bank your wins at every milestone and try simple techniques such as keeping a gratitude journal.

- Small changes become routines that turn into bigger habits, such as one daily press-up leads to 25 which then becomes 1,000 a year, or a daily walk at lunchtime becomes 10,000 steps a day.

- You're a human being not a robot, so don't let one glass of wine derail you or make you cut yourself off from the world. Instead, deal with temptation in social settings by opting for an extra portion of protein-packed chicken and, if desperate, ditch that carb-heavy bread roll that houses your protein.

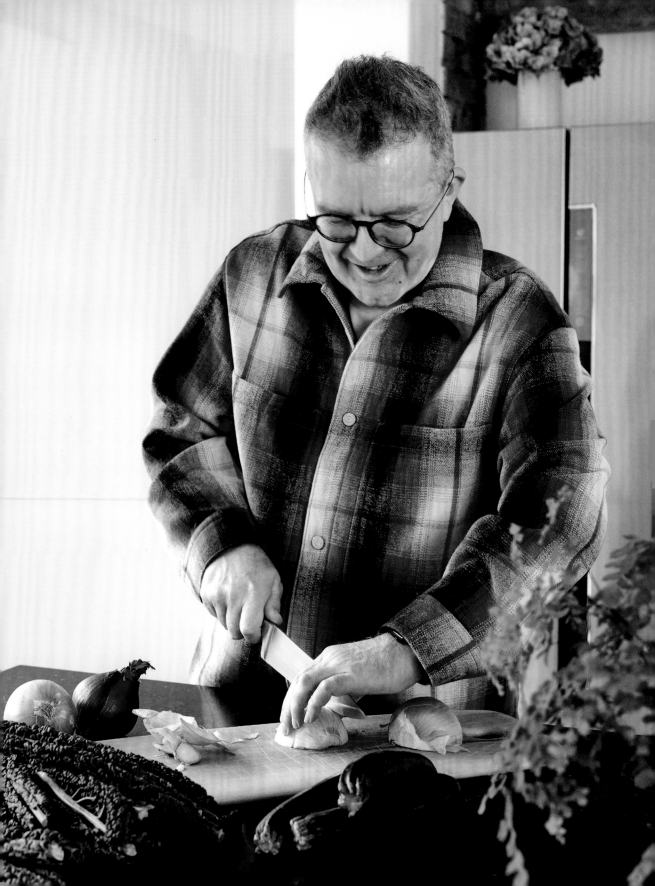

2 Diets

From low-carb to Mediterranean, there are many different types of weight-management diets and what works for one person may not for another. This isn't a diet book, so I'm not going to tell you what you should and shouldn't eat, but in this chapter I'll outline the basic facts about the eating plans I followed. Some may be contradictory. Try attending a conference on nutritional science – no one there would agree! Most modern approaches, though, are based around the proportion of carbohydrate and fat on your plate, and reducing the sugar content. You'll need to decide what works for you and your body. My own relationship with food was akin to an addict's compulsion towards drugs or alcohol. Cutting down a bit for a while wouldn't work. Instead, I had to be brutally honest and face up to the fact it was a *lifetime decision*.

There are some basic principles and strategies that helped me trim down and hopefully you'll get results from them too. Especially if you're at risk of type 2 diabetes or have a diagnosis. Two of the most important are:

- **Eat real meals.** This means nothing processed or microwaved, and don't eat any meal delivered to your house that you don't know what's in it. Better still, don't order takeaways.

- **Avoid empty calories.** These are foods that give you no nutritional benefit, and after eating them your body will be begging for proper sustenance, which leads to cravings and erratic (and toxic) eating habits.

For 30 years, I felt hungry constantly because much of what I ate was of limited nutritional value. Like the pizza after late-night voting in the Commons. Or the chocolate bars I was always on the hunt for, like a person with an addiction searching for the next fix. Eating proper food has saved me, and my body, from the foods that give you a quick energy hit but nothing more. It's also important to:

- **Record what you eat.** Make a note in your diary, notebook or smart phone. Whatever works for you. This may make frightening reading at first. I was in denial for decades before I could bring myself to face what I was really consuming and how much. I did say there would be humiliation on the way! But keeping a record makes you conscious of the calorific assault of foods with zero nutrients that are going into your body.

- **Move every hour.** This is key. I discuss this in detail in Chapter 4, but as a minimum, you should shake out your arms and legs and move around for two minutes.

The last but most important step I took was to beat my addiction to sugar. If you're diabetic nearly everyone says go your own way to find what works for you. But the single most important change I made was to cut out refined sugar.

Going sugar-free

In most areas of life, everything in moderation is useful advice. But not when it comes to sugar. That includes sugar in all its 'hidden' forms: in yogurt, baked beans and sauces such as tomato ketchup. Sugar even lurks in breakfast cereal – an estimated 40% of children's sugar intake comes from breakfast foods, and even 'healthy' muesli contains the sweet stuff in the form of dried fruit. Just because you don't add it, that doesn't mean you're not eating it.

The 'white stuff' provides none of the essential nutrients needed to heal wounds, boost the immune system and keep your bones healthy, such as vitamins, minerals and protein. It contains only calories. In his book *Pure, White and Deadly*, British nutritionist John Yudkin wrote that sugar would be a banned substance if we'd known about its chemical composition.

Sucrose is the name for refined sugar and is made of glucose and fructose. When you eat white sugar, enzymes in the mouth break it down into these two water-soluble compounds. The fructose is processed by the liver and when you eat too much sucrose, the liver cannot process the fructose fast enough. The consequence is that the body carries fructose in the blood. Too much glucose also raises blood sugar levels, which can be dangerous for people with diabetes.

Sugar's link to obesity is also well documented and widely acknowledged. Eating too much can make you gain weight, and this can lead to heart disease and type 2 diabetes. Being overweight can also increase the risk of being seriously ill with COVID-19. I wasn't always fat, especially not as a teenager. The side effects of eating too much sugar creep up on you over time, like obesity.

And sugar is not just playing havoc with your body. It plays havoc with your brain, too, which lights up like a Christmas tree. When sugar lands on your tongue, receptors on your taste buds sense sweetness. This sends a signal to your forebrain, which in turn triggers your brain's reward system. You're stimulating the dopamine high that people crave — my mood always soared then crashed after a sugar binge.

In the previous chapter, I touched on the work done by Professor Ciara McCabe on dopamine. For her research, McCabe used chocolate as a tool in an MRI scanner to activate the reward system in humans. What this showed was there may be truth in people declaring themselves chocolate 'cravers'. She found these individuals have stronger responses than others in the brain's 'reward' centre. Genes may play a part in this. Or stress — many of us over-eat to combat anxiety, and a reward suppresses this stress.

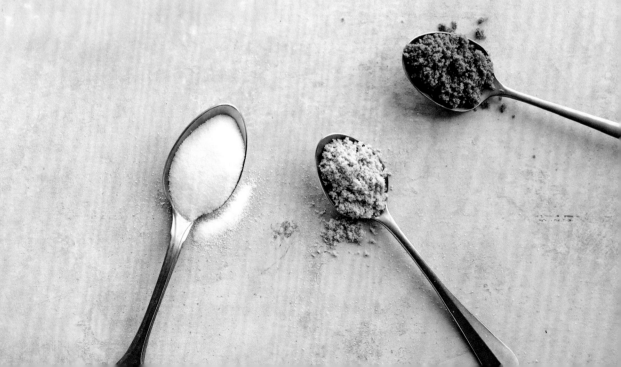

What's being done to reduce sugar in foods?

Around 180 million tonnes of refined sugar is produced each year worldwide. UK consumption rose to nearly 3 million tonnes in 2020, an increase of 3.5% since 2015. A tax was introduced in 2018 on the soft drinks industry in a bid to reduce sugar in drinks and tackle childhood obesity. This has made progress. Sugar content in sugary drinks has fallen 43% over four years according to Public Health England. Other voluntary targets brought in by the UK government have been less successful. A study found that half of companies had not met a 5% reduction goal to lower the amount of sugar in foods by 2018. The results were disappointing for the 2020 target, too: the overall reduction in sugar in products sold was only 3%, well below the 20% set.

The link between sugar and diabetes

Sugary foods and drinks contain a lot of calories. And if you take in more calories than your body needs then you put on weight. Obesity can make your body 'resistant' to the hormone insulin. Made by the pancreas, insulin allows cells to absorb glucose and lowers blood sugar levels. But in obese people, insulin can struggle to do this job properly so blood sugar levels become too high. Type 2 diabetes can result from this. A long-term condition, diabetes can damage the kidneys along with other organs and costs the NHS an estimated £10 billion a year to treat. The most recent figures for 2021 are beginning to show the long-term consequences of Covid on our weight and health. The UK National Child Measurement Programme shows that children entering reception classes in primary schools have seen a 10 per cent increase in obesity in a year.

Just like drugs of abuse, sugar can alter the dopamine receptors to increase the amount of the feel-good hormone released. The good news is that the brain can go back to normal. It's three years now since I last ate milk chocolate, which was among my sweet fixes. Saying 'No' to sugar resulted in me losing 100lb (45.4kg) in less than 12 months. That was nearly a third of my bodyweight.

Whole communities can be transformed, too. In the ITV documentary *Giving Up Sugar: For Good?* I reported on a project by staff at Tameside and Glossop Integrated Care NHS Foundation Trust. They were set a challenge to give up refined sugar. Fizzy drinks and other high-sugar foods were removed from the canteen and the sugar content in meals was reduced as part of the wellbeing drive. The results were jaw-dropping, with some staff losing up to 6 stone (38kg) in weight. Three years on, the hospital is continuing to provide healthier foods to support balanced diets.

How much sugar is in your favourite drink?

250ml glass of dry white wine
sugar = 1.5g
carbs = 4g

A pint of beer
sugar = 0
carbs = 17.6g

A glass of vodka, soda and slice of fresh lime
sugar = 0
carbs = 0

Sugar contains only calories and none of the essential nutrients needed to keep us healthy.

Swapping to low-sugar alcohol

It's not just food that's high in sugar, it's also present in alcohol such as beer and wine. Before downsizing, I drank a lot. There was always a party or reception to go to. And that usually meant liberal amounts of booze. Then I started my weight-loss journey. The question was whether to quit alcohol altogether or to rethink what I poured into my glass. After doing my research, I decided to swap my favourite tipples for drinks that were lower in sugar and in carbs. This meant switching from wine and beer to spirits with no calorie mixers.

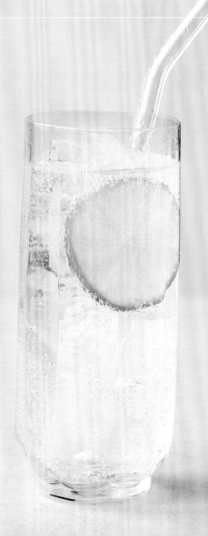

The facts about fat

Remember eating butter as a kid? No one batted an eyelid or warned you it was the path to obesity. We fried with it, lavished it on toast and even ate it mixed with sugar as a treat (weird, I know). Then butter became the poster boy for 'bad' – or saturated – fat.

For the last 30 years, conventional dietary/health advice has told us to reduce our saturated fat intake. Very influential global institutions such as the American Heart Association advised people to reduce their consumption of saturated fat. The recommendation to reduce saturated fat, however, is based mainly on observational studies and is now contested. Advocates of low-carb nutrition argue that most systematic reviews of randomised controlled trials, the strongest type of scientific evidence, do not prove a link between saturated fat and heart disease and the role played by natural saturated fats in a healthy diet is now being reconsidered. Having read a lot on this subject, I don't think the case that saturated fat leads to heart disease has been proven.

Yet for the last three decades, many weight-loss regimes have been based around cutting back on fatty foods. The theory is fats are twice as calorific as carbs, so cutting down on them leads to a slimmer you. Yet some doctors now argue fats have unjustly been given a bad press. Cardiologist Dr Aseem Malhotra says sugar and too many carbohydrates are the enemy, not fat. In fact, he wrote an article to this effect in the esteemed *British Medical Journal*. Malhotra's argument is that obesity is the result of the body storing fat from the overproduction of insulin from carbs.

What's more, some countries, such as Norway and Denmark, have fat-rich diets but heart disease is low. Conversely, people in Chile eat little fat yet have a high rate of heart disease. The Swedish Council on Health Technology did a review involving 16 scientists that concluded that a high-fat, low-carb diet was best for weight loss. They also found this approach helped reduce cardiovascular risk in the obese.

As you can see, the experts are divided. The exception in all of this is trans fats, which are found in processed foods such as cakes. Trans fats are considered such a health risk that many countries, including the US, have banned them. In the UK there's a voluntary agreement with food companies to reduce their use.

I no longer fear saturated fat, though you'll have to make up your own mind about it. Wherever you end up in the debate around fats, I think there is a general consensus that 'good' monounsaturated and polyunsaturated fats are heart-friendly. We're talking olive oil, oily fish such as mackerel and salmon, as well as the fats in some nuts, such as walnuts, and avocados.

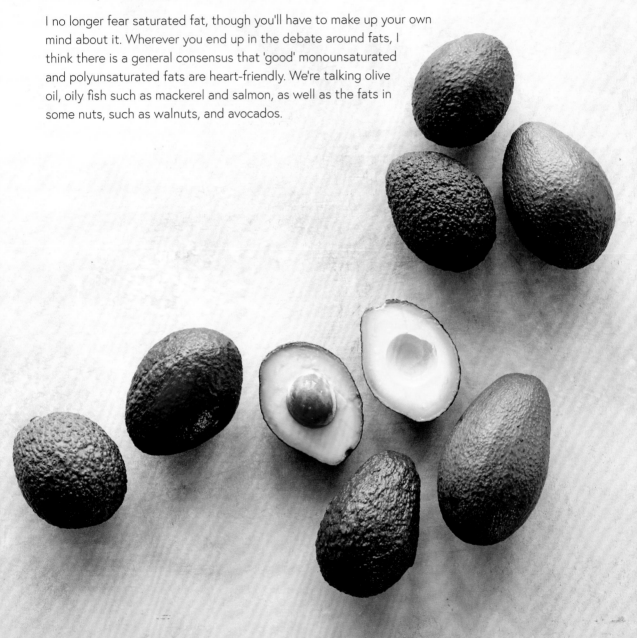

The Western diet

Processed meat, refined grains and lashings of sugar. These are all factory-produced staples of the Western diet, which is to blame for more deaths than smoking and high blood pressure. Our largely urban lifestyles mean we reach for 'convenience' foods – the supermarket ready-meals, the pizza on a Friday night and the inevitable takeaways. These are packed with carbohydrates such as white flour, rice and potato-based chips. The body breaks these down quickly into sugar (glucose), which is released into the bloodstream. But this isn't a good thing. A speedy turnaround results only in a short-lived release of energy, leading to us wanting (and eating) more. And that can pile on the pounds.

What's more, these 'simple' carbs send blood sugar levels soaring. This triggers the pancreas to send out a surge of insulin, which is needed by cells to deal with the glucose, or store it for future use. In the long term, this constant over-reaction isn't good for health. Refined carbs are also often lacking in fibre, an essential aid to digestion and in lowering blood sugar levels. Nor is the high sugar content in a Western diet good for health, as I explained earlier. But the body has no choice except to make use of the energy sources you consume.

How to reinvent chips and fries on a low-carb regime

Chips had been a favourite food. Who doesn't love a bag on the way home from the pub? But note the word 'had'. Once I began downsizing, I realised they were lost to me. There's always hope though. These days I've learned how to make alternatives such as celeriac chips (see page 140) or halloumi chips (see page 147).

Low-carb

What worked for me was a diet based on eating very few carbs. The aim is to cut down the carb content of food to between 20 and 130g a day. Compare this with a typical Western diet, which contains an average of 300g carbs a day – half of the entire energy content you get from food.

In return for carb-cutting, you eat more fat and protein.

So how does it work? Reducing carb consumption makes the body turn to alternative sources of energy. It burns the fat it has stored because it doesn't have enough of the glucose that's produced from breaking down carbohydrates. By getting rid of its fat stocks, the body rapidly loses weight. You've probably heard of the Atkins diet. Invented in 1972 by cardiologist Robert Atkins, this is a low-carb eating plan.

Fasting

Intermittent fasting for weight loss is essentially an eating pattern that switches between periods of not eating and consuming food. So, what's the theory behind it? Your body goes into starvation mode (see the box on metabolism, page 53) which forces your body to use up all its sugar stores. Once these are depleted, it has no choice but to switch to burning fat. This approach has similarities to the ketogenic diet (see page 52). Fasting also increases levels of a protein (BDNF factor) that activates the body's rest and digest response. This can lower blood pressure by reducing heart contractions.

As long as you don't eat between meals, there's no food to process and store. As a result, the pancreas doesn't need to release insulin to help cells absorb glucose, insulin levels go down and fat cells release their stored sugar to be used as energy. Weight loss (in the form of fat burn off) occurs if insulin levels go down far enough and for long enough.

Dr Michael Mosley made fasting popular in his book *The Fast Diet*. Another expert is Canadian Dr Jason Fung, who has a special interest in obesity and diabetes. A kidney specialist and author of *The Diabetes Code*, he suggests patients cut out food for 24 hours, two or three times a week, or for 16 hours, five to six times a week. Nutritionists believe the timing of when you fast may be key to fasting success. The 16:8 diet restricts eating and drinking to an 8-hour daily window, for example from noon to 8pm. Outside these hours your body should be a food-and-drink-free temple.

A study in 2019 said a fasting diet may limit several risk factors for developing cardiovascular diseases and therefore the occurrence of these diseases. However, the research also warned that fasting is not recommended for some people. That includes anyone with a hormonal imbalance, as well as pregnant and breastfeeding women. Moreover, people with eating disorders, a low BMI (under 18.5), and underweight people are also not recommended to try this form of eating. So, before you try fasting, I strongly advise you speak to your doctor first if you're in any of these categories.

Ketogenic

Then there's the ketogenic – or 'keto' – diet. This what I adopted at the start of my downsizing programme, and it helped me shed 2 stone (13kg) in two months. Strict keto is essentially an extreme version of low-carb. By drastically reducing your carbohydrate intake, your body is deprived of them and 'learns' to burn fat instead of carbs to make energy. The carb content in food is largely replaced with fat, for example butter and non-industrially produced oils (avocado, coconut, etc).

Like many eating plans, keto isn't new. The concept originated in the 1920s for children with drug-resistant epilepsy and is still used today in medical care.

As the drastic reduction in carbohydrates needs to be replaced with fats, you must make your own decision on the science around fats. I decided that the weight loss on keto was so effective that it was the best choice for me. At the time, the keto diet was not particularly popular or understood. These days more people have followed this approach to dieting. Beware of some of the myths around keto, though. I've heard too many people say that on a keto diet, the more fat you eat, the more fat you will lose. No, no, no! If you eat more fat than you need for energy, it will slow down your weight loss, even if you have virtually eliminated carbs.

Foods you can eat on keto
- Meat, including poultry
- Fish
- Dairy
- Oils
- Vegetables

Foods that are banned (essentially carbs)
- Pasta
- Rice
- Grains
- Potatoes
- Highly processed convenience foods

I've already talked about bulletproof coffee (see page 34), which is a staple for tackling cravings on keto. Other typical meal options are:

- Bacon and eggs
- Halloumi chips
- Cauliflower cheese
- Spiced salmon
- Steak with broccoli and cauliflower
- Cheese with celery

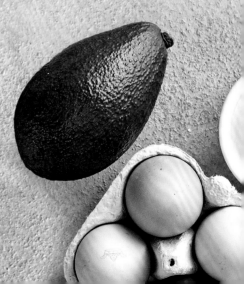

Side effects or withdrawal symptoms – dubbed 'keto flu' – can be an issue with a low-carb/high-fat approach. Initially, I experienced the sensation that I was about to come down with a cold, but it didn't last long. Another potential downside of cutting out the carbs is a lack of fibre, which isn't great for your bowels and is a cancer risk. The key is to eat fibre-rich vegetables (and keep the skin on where possible), such as carrots, beetroot and broccoli. On any low-carb option, you're going to have to find a love of cauliflower and broccoli!

A small-scale study published in 2017 found that people on a sustained ketogenic diet with no exercise lost more weight and body fat compared with those on a standard diet or who exercised 3–5 days a week.

How human metabolism works

Metabolism is the term given to chemical reactions in the body's cells that change food into energy. Nutrition is a key part of this process. The three metabolic states the body switches between on any given day (or night) are:

- **Fed (absorption)** – digesting food after a meal
- **Fasting (post-absorptive)** – all nutrients from food have been digested, absorbed and stored
- **Starvation** – the body's been deprived of nourishment for a time and goes into survival mode

In starvation mode, the body must still provide the brain with fuel to function. First, it uses up its stores of glucose (glycogen). Then it switches to breaking down fat (stored fatty acids) for an alternative fuel source. This process is called ketosis. The fatty acids are converted in the liver into compounds known as ketones, which are released into the blood to fuel the brain and muscles.

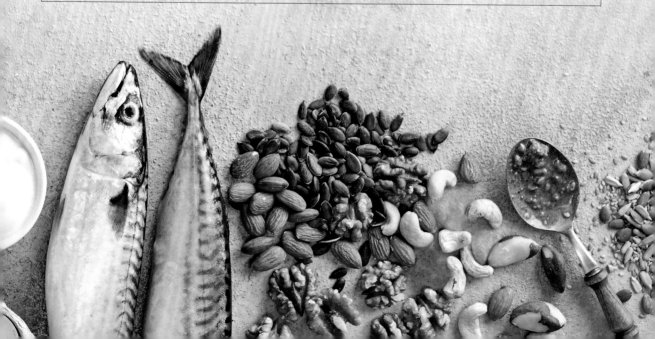

Re-engineering the English breakfast

In the past, families would sit down to protein-packed cockles, mussels and kippers in the morning. Not sugary cereals. Eggs are a rich source of protein, so with this in mind, my breakfast 'makeover' switched from two bowls of Weetabix or two slices of toast with jam washed down with coffee to either: scrambled eggs with smoked salmon, a cheese omelette or bacon and eggs.

Egg-sential facts

One medium-sized egg contains:

- 66 calories

- 5.2g protein

- Iron

- Selenium and iodine

- Vitamins A, B and D

- 4.6g fat (including 1.3g saturates, 1.7g monosaturates, 0.7g polyunsaturates)

Cracking eggs

When I embarked on my low-carb diet, all I knew was that I'd need lots of eggs. It was the first time I'd bought them in cartons of a dozen (rather than six). Eggs were a staple of my diet growing up. That's partly thanks to the now iconic 1965 advertising campaign 'Go to work on an egg' – a slogan attributed to Fay Weldon, who went on to become a bestselling fiction author. Over the years, eggs have remained essential to a traditional English breakfast, but they have fallen in and out of favour with health experts.

There's hardly any fat in the white of an egg; the yolk, however, contains cholesterol, a fatty substance also found in your blood. That's why eggs have been maligned as more evidence has emerged about the links between cholesterol and heart disease. But there's no proven link between *consuming* cholesterol and an increased risk of cardiac problems. The guidance from Heart UK is that eggs don't appear to raise cholesterol levels the way foods containing trans fats do. As I keep saying, this is not a diet book.

All I know is that I've got eggs to thank (among other foods) for my dramatic weight loss. Previously, I'd tuck into a bowl of porridge. That's before I discovered instant oats had a high glycaemic load (more of this later in the book) that was making my blood sugar fluctuate and putting me on the path to full-blown type 2 diabetes. And what's better is that eggs are sugar-free, unlike breakfast cereals, which are packed with the sweet stuff.

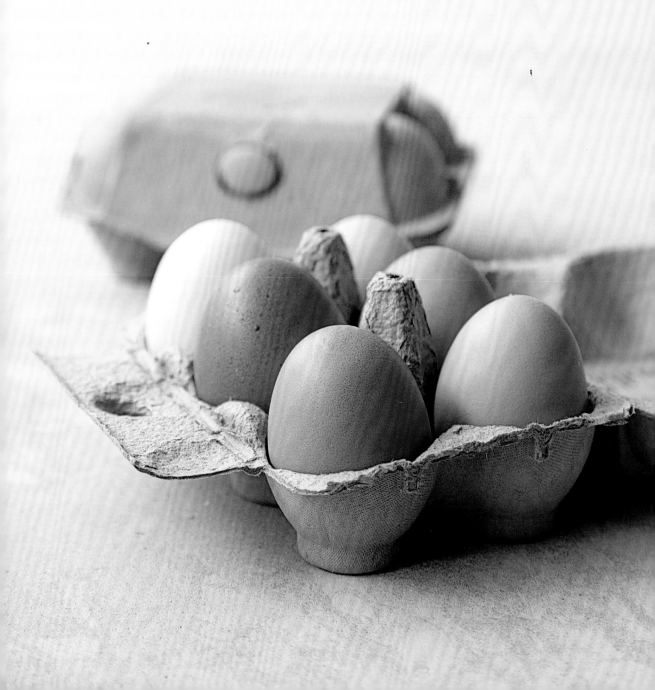

Eggs are a rich source
of protein – and
they're sugar-free.

Studies show that
a Mediterranean
diet reduces the risk
of sudden cardiac
death (SCD).

Mediterranean

As you travel on your weight-loss journey you'll discover which ways of eating suit you best.

Keto produced dramatic results for me. After a while, though, I decided to move on to a more balanced approach, one that can be loosely described as a Mediterranean diet.

I'm sure you've seen stories about places in Greece and Italy where everyone lives to a hundred, can still run up mountains and has the blood pressure of a 30-year-old, and it's true their excellent health is largely down to their style of eating and what they eat. Again, this is typically a diet low in sugar and starchy carbohydrates. Any carbs tend to come not from processed foods but from unrefined foods that are rich in fibre, such as beans and whole wheat. The fat content for this eating plan is moderate. It usually comes from healthy unsaturated oils such as (monounsaturated) olive oil. A Mediterranean diet is also rich in nuts, vegetables, seeds and fish, which are all packed with polyunsaturated fats.

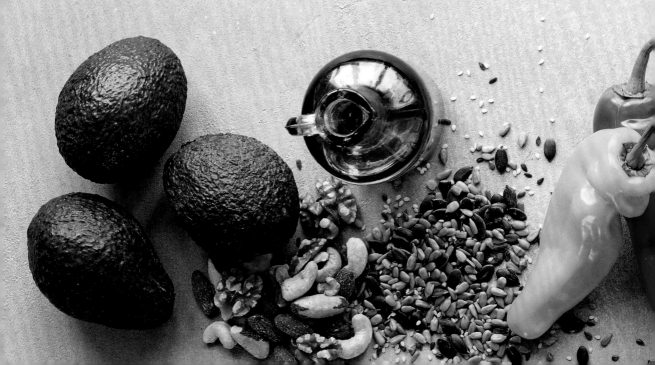

For me, this way of eating meant tins of tuna and mackerel fillets as a source of protein. Combined with a mixed salad, these fish treats were a tasty snack and helped curb cravings. Of course, it's important to bear in mind that people in many Mediterranean countries are also more active, have regular meal patterns (rather than grabbing a sandwich on the go) and supportive social networks. These factors all help too.

But there are numerous published studies that conclude a diet rich in unsaturated fats and oily fish has many health benefits. These include a reduction in the risk of heart disease and developing diabetes.

The secret to longevity

A coastal village on the Tyrrhenian Sea, Pioppi has been recognised by UNESCO as being the home of the Mediterranean diet. The inhabitants of this southern Italian village are also said to have a longer life expectancy. On average, it's close to ninety and many live to over a hundred. Cardiologist Dr Aseem Malhotra and documentary maker Donal O'Neill were so inspired by the place that they named their low-carb eating *The Pioppi Diet* in recognition of it.

Research published in 2021 based on more than 20,000 people showed a Mediterranean diet reduced the likelihood of sudden cardiac death (SCD). This is a condition where your heart stops pumping blood around your body without warning and is the largest cause of natural death in the US. Those who said they ate a Mediterranean-style diet were less at risk of SCD than those who ate foods such as fried foods, processed meats and sugar-sweetened drinks.

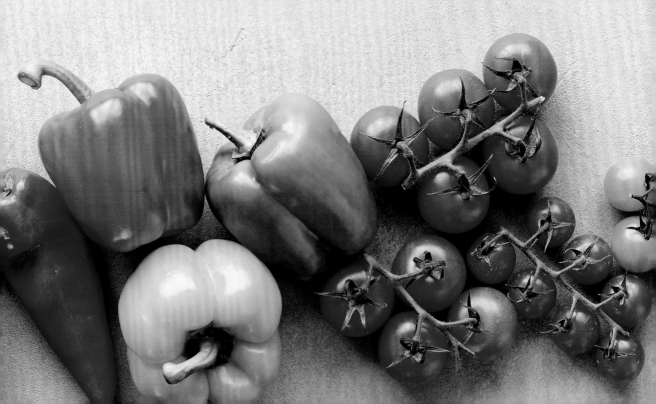

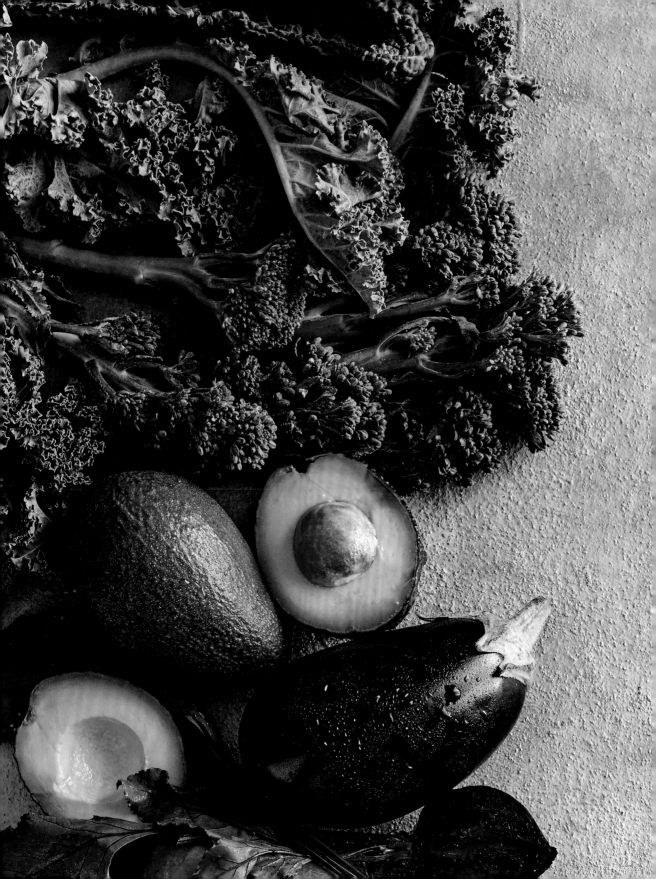

- A Western diet is packed with refined sugar and too little fibre, so avoid meals with zero nutritional benefit and switch to real food, especially if you're type 2 diabetic.

- Fat isn't the enemy.

- Cutting carb intake makes the body burn fat and this often leads to weight loss.

- A ketogenic diet can shed the weight but can be fibre-light – counteract this by eating lots of vegetables, such as broccoli and cauliflower.

- Eat like an Italian by having varied meals that are rich in vegetables, olive oil and healthy nuts – people in the Italian town Pioppi are long-lived and have less chance of a sudden cardiac arrest.

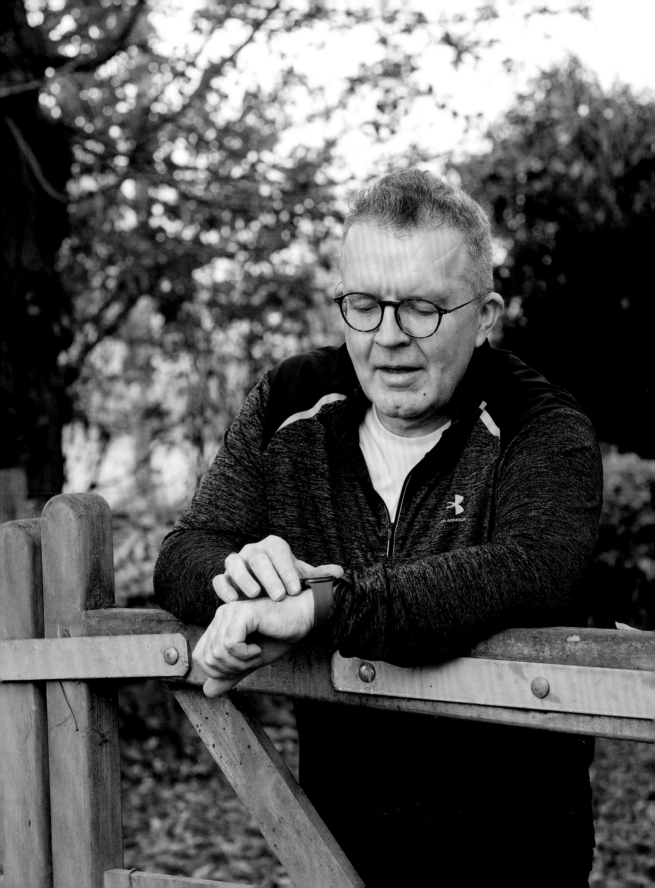

3 Measurement

An essential part of downsizing is measuring on a daily basis – not only your weight but factors related to this, such as blood sugar levels and blood pressure. The current marker widely used by doctors for working out if your weight is healthy or not is body mass index (BMI). This is basically your weight adjusted for height. In the next few pages, I'll discuss whether BMI is a useful way of telling how healthy you are. We'll also look at why it's important to maintain steady blood sugar levels. It was a chance meeting with a doctor at a party that led to my type 2 diabetes diagnosis. As a result of this bombshell revelation, I followed a very specific weight-loss programme but the basics can be applied to everyone, whether they are diabetic or have high blood pressure or just want to downsize.

An estimated 36%
of adults in the UK
are overweight.

Carrying excess pounds – or an extra 8 stone (50.8kg) in my case – is a red flag for a range of issues including type 2 diabetes. A series of punishing lockdowns over the past year or more have added to our woes by playing havoc with our routines and leaving many of us larger than we'd like to be. The doors to the gym and leisure centres were bolted for what seemed forever, and even those fortunate enough to be near green spaces ended up bored with pacing around the same patch of turf every day.

The need for a lifestyle reset triggered by the pandemic may even be the reason you're reading this book now. A nationwide survey commissioned by Public Health England and published in July 2021 found that 41% of the nation's adults said they had put on weight since the first lockdown in March 2020. Snacking and comfort eating were the major culprits, which isn't surprising given we were forced to stay at home within easy reach of the fridge and kitchen cupboards.

You may have had the opposite experience and found you've piled on the pounds since returning to work. The temptations of that pasty at lunch from the café within walking distance, of the office biscuit tin or that cappuccino with a croissant on the way into the office may well have set you back in the weight stakes. That's when you become fearful of stepping on the scales.

Those at high risk of type 2 diabetes have been particularly vulnerable to the impact of lockdowns. A study suggests that during the pandemic there may have been an increase in bodyweight for people who are highly likely to develop the disease. The researchers found that those who signed up during 2020 and the start of 2021 to an NHS diabetes prevention programme were 5lb (2.4kg) heavier than people who joined in the three years before 2020.

I too struggled during stay-at-home restrictions. At my lowest point during those bleak and oppressive months, I even began to wonder if I'd lost control. Was 'big fat Tom' on the way back? The very thought of slipping back to the unhealthy person I once was terrified me. My response was to reapply some rules, which I will outline in more detail later. And what I learned is that you can retrace your steps to find the right path again. It just takes a reboot, a return to the downsizing 'settings' I've outlined in this book, such as refocusing on changing behaviour, banking new wins and paying attention to what you're putting in your mouth by eating real, not processed, food. Getting a proper sleep is crucial too – I can't stress the importance of this enough and always found I weighed less on the scales when I'd had a full night's rest.

Even with a reset, successive enforced lockdowns were tough for me. My routines and habits were smashed. I spent more of my time being sedentary and closer to the food cupboard. Though I didn't return to the bad old days of high-sugar foods and microwave meals, I did succumb to new temptations.

The disaster for me was cheese. It wasn't until I read *Fork in the Road – a hopeful guide to food freedom* by Dr Jen Unwin that I realised it is widespread for former sugar addicts to fixate on a new food type, very often cheese. It just goes to show that maintaining weight loss always throws up new challenges to overcome.

Reversing type 2 diabetes

The science behind Dr Mosley's rapid weight-loss approach to reversing type 2 diabetes is based on research by Roy Taylor. A hospital consultant and expert at Newcastle University, Professor Taylor performed a study that showed type 2 diabetes is caused by fat accumulating in the pancreas – and that losing less than 1g of fat in the pancreas through weight reduction reverses the deadly disease. The only way to achieve this is by calorie restriction, he concluded, whether by diet or an operation. His work transformed the thinking on type 2 diabetes as this was the first time that it had been demonstrated that diet could remove the fat clogging up the pancreas and allow normal insulin secretion to be restored. He found that regardless of present bodyweight and how you lose weight, the critical factor in reversing type 2 diabetes is losing that 1g of fat from the pancreas. Professor Taylor's study was later used as the basis for a more comprehensive trial, which found that almost half of people put on a diet of fewer than 900 (825–53) calories a day for up to five months achieved remission after a year and were able to come off medication.

Challenging the Eatwell guidance

A word here about the Eatwell 'plate'. You may have heard of this or perhaps your doctor might have recommended using one if you're trying to lose weight. It's essentially a pie chart divided into segments which each represent a food group and how much you should eat from each group every day. The proportions are based on the government's recommendations in order to achieve a balanced diet. After my diabetes diagnosis in 2013, I was referred to a nutritionist to sort out my poor eating choices (including two cheeseburgers in one go) which had contributed to my ever-expanding waistline and constant fatigue. What she explained to me was that the Eatwell guidelines recommended five portions of fruit and vegetables daily along with starchy carbs such as rice, and that fat (especially saturated) should be reduced as well as foods high in sugar.

As a consequence I started to measure my portion sizes using a small pair of kitchen scales, as the nutritionist suggested, and cut back on cake and biscuit treats. An awareness of temptations and how they affected me also began to kick in. For this, I'm grateful. Yet despite following the Eatwell guidance my weight did not budge, which was a major source of frustration for me. This is when I began doing my own research and high on my list was Dr Michael Mosley's *The 8-Week Blood Sugar Diet*, which advocates a low-calorie, low-carb, Mediterranean-style eating programme (see page 56) to combat type 2 diabetes.

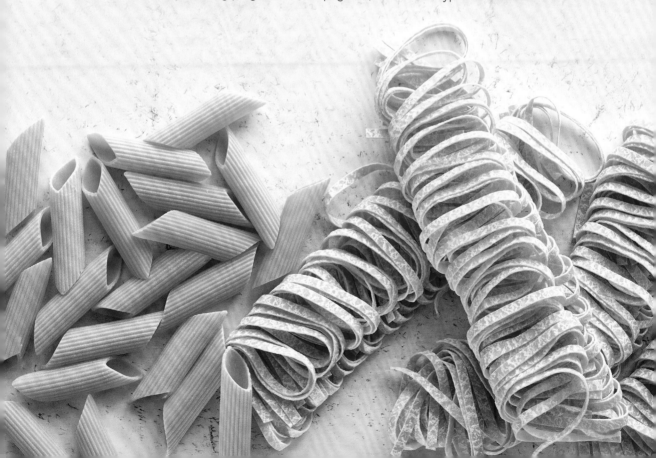

Ditching pasta, bread and rice altogether – or at least consuming them in tiny quantities – was not what the Eatwell guidance advised. What's more, Mosley recommended a diet rich in full-fat dairy and eggs. I'm not saying the Eatwell approach wasn't helpful in opening my eyes to my unhealthy eating patterns, adopting its guidance may even enable some readers to downsize, but for me Eatwell didn't work and that's why I ended up moving on from this dietary approach and following another path. And the Eatwell advice, which is essentially to eat carbs in order to get healthy, is not sensible for people who have type 2 diabetes and may even do them harm. As soon as I recognised that, I started to get well.

The evidence in front of my own eyes has taught me that every food you eat will impact differently on every individual's blood sugar level and on their body in general. We are all unique. Not everyone's body can handle the amount of carbohydrates the Eatwell guide recommends. The one-size-fits-all policy behind Eatwell came along before technology allowed us to measure what food we put inside ourselves. That's why Public Health England (PHE) had not caught up with the freedom technology gives us to create our own tailored downsizing programmes. A more personalised approach is vital for treating people with diabetes, and GPs should get more training in nutrition so they can better support patients. This failure may be why, in 2021, PHE was replaced by a new body called the Office for Health Improvement and Disparities (OHID). The test for success will be whether it can provide personal health advice to people seeking to downsize.

Quantify your downsizing

What worked for me was to 'gamify' my weight loss, in other words to apply elements such as measurements, scores, goals and rules to keep me on track. As a kid who grew up with console video games, I just applied the same strategies that helped me win then to achieving weight loss. It was about starting small but thinking big. The daily details of every meal, including calorie content, were recorded in MyFitnessPal app that tracks your progress. Alternatively, jot down the results in a notebook, if pen and paper works better for you.

Knowing how many calories is in that energy bar or tub of hummus and the result of your daily weigh-in can be alarming at first, especially if you've been in denial for years. Although it's brutal, facing up to the truth was a major turning point for me – I started to take control. Advances in technology mean apps and fitness devices will do the maths for you and provide you with data you can access instantly on your progress in the short and long term. With MyFitnessPal you can even scan a barcode and find out exactly what you're eating down to the last nutrient. Use these apps as you would a true friend to support and guide you as you live, hour by hour in the early stages, then day by day, then week by week. Or on reset when it's necessary to go back to setting a target for tomorrow.

Habits lead to change

In the early days, measuring results and outcomes is helpful in laying down habits on which you can rely when faced with temptation or boredom. Once you've embedded these routines then your subconscious should guide you. It's like learning a recipe – the first few times you stick rigidly to the method and ingredients, but once you've practised enough you know how much you need and how to put it all together.

These days I don't look at how many daily steps I've done, unless I need to do a reset. You'll know when to do this. There are the tell-tale signs. Are your clothes feeling tight? Do you have brain fog? Are you feeling sluggish? You may not be regularly measuring your weight but are periodic readings heading in the wrong direction?

When the signs indicate you need a reset, the good habits you've fixed firmly in your brain become invaluable.

Laying down deep habits is complicated. It goes to the core of how you see yourself, who you are. If you can become the person who is active, not slothful, the person that always takes the stairs, not the escalator, you'll get back on track. Writing your own story – and believing it – is why habits are powerful tools in your downsizing journey.

It was the same with following an eating plan. I've outlined how I started off following a strict keto diet, where you're limited to less than 50g of carbs a day (an average apple contains 25g), but after a while I was able to relax this regime and allow in more carbs. This is a practice known as keto 'cycling', where you have a day or more on which you allow carbs into your daily eating regime. It's not an excuse to go crazy and binge on biscuits or cakes, the aim is to allow yourself a higher carb intake on 'refeeding days' to replenish your glucose stores and make it easier to stick to the overall keto plan. The prospect of a rule-relaxation day makes you more motivated to be strict the rest of the time.

To lose 8 stone (50.8kg) was the long-term goal I set myself at the start of my journey. I succeeded by breaking down this task into small steps so that it wasn't too daunting. Having a sense of where you want to be in a week, a month or a year gives you a finish line to cross. Weight loss isn't a competition, though, or a race. It's more like an expedition with both setbacks and triumphs along the way, which is why to reach and *maintain* your target you need to start off with daily measuring and monitoring. As I headed out of the house, I'd know my weight and blood sugar level and would have logged my first meal of the day on my app. And this would give the knowledge and focus I needed to handle whatever life had in store for me. The lows, as well as the highs.

How to change behaviour and habits

According to author James Clear, there are three levels at which change occurs and which enable you to stick to your goals. In his book, *Atomic Habits*, he likens them to the layers of an onion. The first layer is Outcome, which is largely associated with the goals you set, for example, losing weight. Then there's Process Change – how you change your habits/systems, such as implementing a new routine at the gym. The deepest layer is Identity. To build a new image for yourself, you need to change your world view and beliefs about yourself, to identify the person you want to become for this to happen. In my case, I wanted to become the person who moved more. Most people just focus on what they want to achieve, but Clear's view is that you need all three levels to achieve lasting success. And to use a reward system – or 'small wins' – to motivate yourself, for example, by buying a pedometer to record the fact that you're more active.

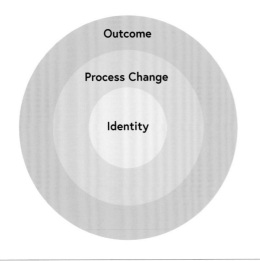

Outcome

Process Change

Identity

800 million people worldwide are obese.

A healthy balance

I briefly touched on the term 'metabolism' earlier (see page 53). It's the process by which your body converts food and drink into energy, the fuel that keeps us going (and alive) on a daily basis.

Metabolic rate is the speed at which your body burns calories to release energy. Then there's metabolic *health*, which is defined as having the right levels of blood sugar and 'good' fats (high-density lipoprotein or HDL) vs 'bad' (low-density lipoprotein – LDL – and triglycerides).

The tell-tale signs of metabolic syndrome

- Extremely overweight or too much fat around the waist

- High triglyceride and low HDL levels in the blood

- High blood pressure (consistently above 140mmHg, over 90mmHg or higher)

- An inability to control blood sugar levels

Healthy blood pressure and normal waist circumference are also markers for metabolic health. With the right lifestyle choices and eating approach, it's possible to be metabolically 'fit' without the need to resort to medications.

Why is metabolic health such a hot issue? If your blood pressure, blood sugar levels, waist circumference and cholesterol (HDL) are not within normal ranges then you're more likely to end up in hospital or dying early. The medical term for a combination of all these risk factors *together* is metabolic 'syndrome', which sends you to the top of the danger list. As well as diabetes, it increases your chances of developing other obesity-related illnesses such as heart disease and stroke. And having see-sawing blood sugar levels leaves you trapped in a cycle of highs and lows – a steep increase in blood sugar is followed by a crash, which in turn triggers hunger pangs. Cue what used to be me reaching for the nearest snack to compensate. Feelings of dizziness, disorientation and brain fog had become so much a part of my life that I didn't question them. It was only later that I came to realise these 'zoning out' episodes were probably due to my blood sugar levels plummeting dangerously low. This is commonly referred to as a 'hypo', or diabetes-related hypoglycaemia.

There's even evidence that other conditions, such as dementia, are linked to metabolic health. A study published in 2020 found that metabolic syndrome increased the risk of vascular dementia, a condition caused by decreased blood flow to the brain that is often as a result of small strokes. What the research also found was that metabolic syndrome is associated with Alzheimer's. Improvements in metabolic syndrome can reduce dementia symptoms, the researchers found.

> See-sawing blood sugar levels leaves you trapped in a cycle of highs and lows.

The stark reality is that 800 million people worldwide are living with obesity and experts warn that current approaches are failing. A call to action published in *The Lancet* medical journal highlighted the need for obesity to be recognised as a disease and health issue, and for metabolic health to become a priority post-pandemic. Excess body fat has even been blamed for worse outcomes for patients infected with COVID-19 and increased severity of symptoms. In blunt terms, the message is: the fatter you are, the more chance you have of becoming very sick or not recovering from the virus. One research study, based on data relating to more than 6 million people, found a direct association between excess weight and admission to hospital and to intensive care. If anything is a wake-up call that change is needed, it's the consequences of a pandemic.

The UK government appears to be taking steps to improve the nation's metabolic health. In March 2021, the Department for Health and Social Care created a new Office for Health Promotion, which promises to tackle obesity and promote physical activity. Do governments learn from past failures on tackling obesity though? The answer is 'No', according to an assessment of obesity strategies in England over 30 years, which found that ministers also rely too much on individuals to make behaviour changes. The authors say few policies have focused on external influences such as unhealthy foods, or taken steps to restrict choice, for example banning promotion of crisps or chocolate.

Government policies aside, what is encouraging to know is that we can all learn from our own mistakes. Metabolic syndrome is *reversible* – you can restore your body to a healthy state where it begins to function normally again, as I discovered.

Achieving good metabolic health

Exercise and eating regimes that avoid highly processed foods are the foundations for improving metabolic health and turning the tables on metabolic syndrome. Professor Luigi Fontana, in his book *The Path to Longevity*, points out that health is our most precious asset and we often blame bad genes or bad luck for diseases such as diabetes. In reality, he says, many metabolic disorders are preventable and it's never too late to start living a healthier life. This echoes what I've said throughout this book about commitment and forming healthy habits. Nutrition, exercise, mind training and mindfulness are just some of the ways of following a path that means you may live longer, according to Fontana. He's also a proponent of 5:2 intermittent fasting (see page 51 for the benefits of fasting). But don't think you can feast on bad food then starve yourself – the advice from Fontana is to follow a diet of fibre-rich vegetables. He's in favour of a largely plant-based diet that's minimally processed with some fasting, as followed by the long-lived residents of Sardinia. Movement, physical activity (that means looking after animals if you're an average Sardinian) and fulfilling social relationships are part of the recipe for success.

Rating carbs: glycaemic index and glycaemic load

The roller-coaster effect of fluctuating sugar levels can cause dramatic symptoms, which is a sign that you're eating food that's not good for you. And when your levels are high, then shifting the flab is going to be practically impossible. The reason why is that the more you consume carbohydrates, the more glucose there is in your bloodstream, and the more insulin is produced by the body. I've outlined already the relationship between glucose storage and insulin (see page 50), but insulin doesn't just remove glucose from the blood, it also promotes fat storage. With all the extra insulin in your body, you will just keep gaining weight because insulin blocks the release of fat.

For me, a carbohydrate binge such as salt and vinegar crisps would even affect my sight as well as my thinking powers. I'd have to scrunch my eyes up to focus and would be hit with such heavy feelings of lethargy that I was prone to nodding off and afternoon napping. Which doesn't lend itself to leading a more active day or life. What I also hadn't realised was that the carbohydrate content of basmati rice – a food that had been central to my diet for years – was a major culprit for sending my blood sugar soaring. I only discovered this after reading about Dr David Unwin, a GP in Merseyside who has been pioneering a low-carb approach and is credited with successfully inspiring many of his patients to reverse their type 2 diabetes. The catalyst had been a study he undertook to examine how many teaspoons of sugar are in commonly eaten foods. He then based his findings around their glycaemic index (GI), a rating system for foods to determine how rapidly their carb contents raise blood sugar.

First developed in the early 1980s for diabetes patients, GI is based on a general rule that refined and processed carbohydrates release glucose more quickly than foods high in protein, fibre and fat. The index ranks glycaemic foods as low (from 0 to 55), medium (56 to 69) and high (70 to 100). The smaller the number, the slower-acting the food and the less impact on your blood sugar.

High GI	Medium GI	Low GI
• white rice	• banana	• broccoli
• watermelon	• sweet yogurt	• chickpeas
• dried cranberries	• boiled sweet potato	• skimmed milk

Yes, my favourite meal choice of white rice is right up there – it's GI rating is equivalent to 10 teaspoons of sugar according to Dr Unwin's research. The advice from him is simple and straightforward – cut down on foods that are high in sugars and starchy carbs, and increase the intake of leafy green vegetables. By offering his patients alternatives to drugs, his GP practice has potentially saved the NHS £60,000 a year and given people like me their lives back.

The limitations of the GI approach have been highlighted by some critics. These include the fact that foods with a high sugar content – such as ice cream – may have a medium GI score despite being an unhealthy choice. Conversely healthy ones – such as some types of beans – score highly. A high-scoring fruit, for example, is watermelon, although you'd need to eat a lot of it to raise your blood sugar levels significantly.

What's also worth bearing in mind is the GI rating varies according to several factors. The carb content of bananas rises as they ripen, which is down to the starch breaking down and the sugar content increasing. The same occurs in fruits such as strawberries, with the sugars making the berries sweeter. And overcooking pasta can raise the GI value – the longer it's in the pan, the more digestible its starches become and the quicker your body converts its carbs to glucose. Eating it al dente, like the Italians, helps prevent this from happening.

Covid and the human cost of obesity

A study by Tufts University in the US found that 30% of more than 900,000 COVID-19 hospital admissions were related to obesity, more than a quarter (26%) to high blood pressure, more than one in five (21%) to diabetes, and 12% to heart failure. Overall, 64% of COVID-19 hospital admissions were attributable to these four conditions together.

The issue over the usefulness of GI has been addressed by another type of food classification called glycaemic load (GL). What GL does is assess the *amount* of carbs in a food portion as well as how much that will then raise a person's blood glucose level. How you calculate GL is to multiply the GI by the amount of carbohydrate (in grams) in a food serving and then divide the total by 100. If we go back to the watermelon, a 100g serving has a GI of 72 but a GL of just 2.

Whatever the criticism of GI, Dr Unwin has shown how his patients' blood sugar levels are affected through evidence detailed in weekly graphs which link their diet to GI. I also know that GI has been a useful guide in helping me identify foods that affect my blood sugar levels and pointing me on the right path to remission from type 2 diabetes.

Measuring blood sugar levels

If you're concerned about your metabolic health or have type 2 diabetes, then blood sugar management is key. Given I'd taken sugar out of my diet, the aim for me was to ensure that I had rid myself of it, and I came to realise blood sugar levels were as important as weight loss. They're an instant indicator that you're putting the right/wrong stuff into your body.

By measuring your own levels, you become more confident and have less need to visit your doctor (although always do everything in consultation with them). I'd recommend testing your levels with a finger-prick test daily, as I did, to help you make decisions on what foods to eat and which ones to avoid. Or, better still, use a continuous glucose monitor (CGM).

If you're squeamish, you will be imagining big needles and blood oozing everywhere, but the reality is it's a tiny prick in your finger and nothing to fear. You just put the drop of blood on to a test slip which then goes into a small gadget called a glucose monitor (it resembles a pedometer). This then comes up with a reading, which appears on the screen, showing how much sugar is in your blood.

A few years before my diagnosis, I'd been referred by my GP to a specialist clinic where they devised a special diet programme. The nurse there issued me with a blood sugar/glucose monitor but I was too overwhelmed at the time to summon up the courage to actually open

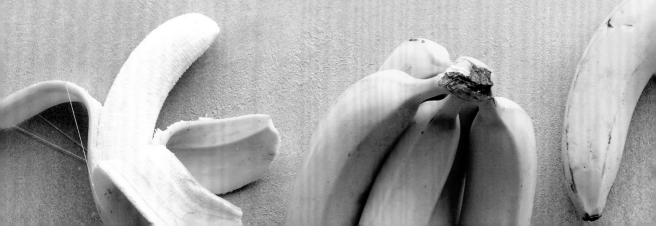

the kit and test myself. Instead, I relied upon the checks done by my doctor, which indicate if your blood sugar levels have been higher than normal on average in the past few months. What the test does is check for how much sugar is in your red blood cells, and it is an important indicator of long-term glycaemic control.

The aim specifically is to look for something called HbA1c (glycated haemoglobin), a protein molecule that's made when the glucose in your body attaches to red blood cells. If your body can't use the glucose properly, then more of it sticks to your cells and builds up in the blood. It was my HbA1c result that confirmed the astonishing news that less than a year after I began my downsizing journey I was back in the normal range. That was according to the official NHS measurement guidelines and meant with a result of 4.9mmol/L that my diabetes had been reversed. I knew it in advance of the test because my regular finger-prick tests began to come down within weeks of me reducing carbohydrates. Yet having the GP tell me that the measurement was in the average range, made it feel official. In consultation with my GP, I was able to start reducing the medication (metformin) I had been prescribed for my diabetes. My success was the result of strictly monitoring and measuring my carbohydrate levels, and it's an outcome that anyone reading this book can achieve. I know if you're reading this, you'll have taken the decision to do something about your health. That's an amazing step in itself. My advice then is to get yourself checked out as soon as you can and start monitoring, because the sooner you do this, the sooner you can get your blood sugar levels down.

Usually, a doctor does your HbA1c score only every 12 months and the downside of this is that it doesn't measure the fluctuations in your conditions between check-ups. By investing in a blood glucose monitor, you get a more accurate sense over time of your blood sugar levels. What's more, you will be able to tell exactly how much sugar is in your body at a particular moment, such as after a meal, so you can gain more control over the food you consume.

That said, a finger-prick test will only give you a snapshot of a couple of minutes a day of what's happening. For a more comprehensive picture, a continuous glucose monitor (CGM) provides readings throughout the day and night so you can track your highs and lows, link these to what you're eating in more detail, and eliminate foods (the bad stuff) that give you a glucose spike. Of course, you're more likely to get one with a can of cola than a portion of

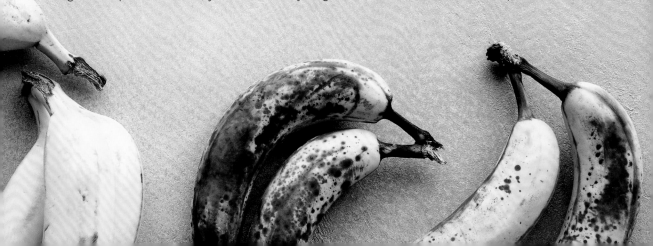

Blood sugar level ranges

When your doctor does a blood glucose test it will be after you've not eaten for at least 8 hours. This enables them to tell how well your body is able to manage blood sugar levels without the influence of food. That's why a fasting glucose measurement is the most important one you can take – you do it before eating breakfast when the body is 'clean' of sugar. Normal blood glucose ranges for people without diabetes are 3.5–5.5 mmol per litre of blood before meals, and less than 8 mmol/L 2 hours after meals. If you have type 2 diabetes, the target is 6–8mmol/L before food or 6–10mmol/L after. Everyone varies, though – I can be either above or below and average around 7% of the time according to the graph I've got on my phone. Do check out www.diabetes.co.uk for more information on blood glucose and monitoring.

cauliflower, but it's still a revelation to see the impact of particular foodstuffs on your unique physiology when you first start monitoring. A pot of yogurt is among the foods that give me a higher spike – don't ask me why, but it does.

You can also witness how long it takes to bring levels back down. If your body can get sugar out of its system more quickly, it suggests better metabolic health.

The thought of wearing a device on your arm may be off-putting. But what we're talking about here is a little plastic disc slightly larger than the diameter of a pound coin which you will hardly notice and is attached to the back of your arm. The disc holds a tiny wire sensor that is inserted under your skin to measure the glucose in the fluid surrounding your cells, and you wear the gadget for two weeks at a time before replacing it with a new one. Some people alternate between arms to give one a rest.

They're not cheap – I bought my starter kit, which gives you 28 days' use, for around £100 – but for me, the investment has been more than worth it. A CGM is a game-changing device that for the first time allows individuals to check their blood sugar highs and lows. I'd go as far as to say it's possibly one of the most revolutionary health technology breakthroughs in 25 years if you've got type 2 diabetes.

When you first use a CGM, it's a diagnostic tool – later on you will come to realise it is also a motivational tool, a way of changing your behaviour. This goes back to what I've said before about using elements of game playing in your weight-loss programme. You go to a coffee shop and feel tempted by the sight of the sugary snack right there in front of you by the till. You think, 'It can't hurt to try it', but your brain is also telling you that you don't want to see that reading come up on your phone. The one that demonstrates the inescapable fact that a lapse has led to a spike in your blood sugar levels which will have inevitable consequences. For the first few weeks and months of monitoring, you'll be listing every item of food you eat and checking the impact on your own body. Once you're familiar with the basics of blood sugar monitoring, you barely need to look at your phone screen to know what will happen. It becomes intuitive. Your body will feel great for a few minutes, then begin to feel shaky. Then comes the slump (in my case, sometimes face down on my desk).

Waist up: BMI

You may be reading this book because your doctor has said your BMI (body mass index) is too high. Based on your weight divided by your height, this measurement is used to calculate where you are on the scale from underweight to obese. A score of over 25 is considered overweight and over 30 is obese.

At my heaviest, with a BMI of 44.1, I was deemed to be at the higher end of the scale. That's a euphemistic way of saying I was extremely obese, so fat that I was even offered weight-loss (bariatric) surgery. I said no on the grounds that it is an invasive procedure, but it was a wake-up call to have reached the point where such a procedure was an option.

The question is how useful is BMI as a measurement? And is it the right benchmark for progress on your downsizing journey? There's a growing feeling among some medical

A gut feeling

Trillions of bacteria, viruses and even fungi live in the gut. Some good, some bad. Together they're known as your gut microbiota or microbiome which has been linked with chronic disease, including type 2 diabetes. Quite how they have an impact is still a work in progress for researchers. The theory is that the microbiome may influence insulin resistance, digestion of sugars and hormones that control this entire process. This is the point where you may be wondering how you can 'measure' your gut bacteria. The answer is you can't, because they're microscopic (although scientists obviously can). However, an unhealthy gut does appear to be related to what you eat –

and a low-carb diet may help overcome this. A study published in 2021 showed that a higher intake of processed foods, alcohol and sugar, corresponds to a microbial environment that is associated with inflammation, and with higher levels inflammatory markers in the intestine. The authors suggest that modulation of gut microbiota through diets enriched in vegetables, legumes, grains, nuts and fish has a potential to prevent intestinal inflammatory processes at the core of many problems such as heart disease. There's growing evidence that type 2 diabetes not only leads to inflammation but precedes the development of the chronic condition.

The history of BMI

In the 1830s, a Belgian astronomer and statistician Lambert Adolphe Jacques Quetelet came up with the theory that the weight of an 'average man' increases in proportion to height. His calculation of body mass divided by height in m² was known as the Quetelet Index and was based on data relating to white men. This was renamed the Body Mass Index in 1972, when physiologist Ancel Keys concluded BMI was the best way of predicting body fat. The World Health Organization then adopted BMI in the 1990s as their standard measure for defining weight, and BMI still remains widely used today.

professionals that BMI is an outdated measurement that doesn't work and needs replacing – or at least modifying. Doctors, other healthcare professionals and even the World Health Organization have relied on BMI for decades to determine healthy bodyweight.

What the evidence is now suggesting is that BMI is misleading among certain populations. If you're Asian, then you can have the same BMI as a white person but have a higher risk of diabetes. The theory is that the associations between BMI, percentage of body fat and health risks are different for Asian populations than those who are from Europe. A study that modified the normal BMI criteria so it took into account the higher percentage of body fat among Asian people and then used the new approach to assess cardiovascular risks among people living in a particular area of India found that high blood pressure was more likely to be predicted and diagnosed (including in the early stages) when body fat percentage was taken into account. This is compared with the standard way of measuring BMI (weight divided by height).

What's also misleading is that BMI won't tell you what proportion of your weight is muscle mass, bone or water. If you're a rugby player or a bodybuilder, then you could end up being defined as having a problem in the weight department when in reality you may be perfectly fit and healthy. Granted, rugby players and bodybuilders make up a tiny percentage of the global population, but if you are very tall you could also fall foul of the BMI calculations.

There needs, therefore, to be a rethink on using BMI as a blanket method of identifying who is at risk. In my view, and in the opinion of some experts, a better measurement would be a

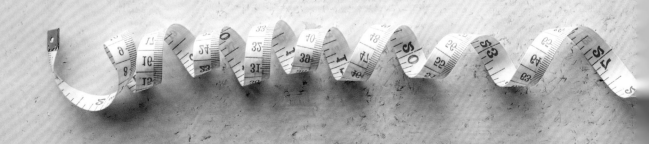

score that includes blood pressure, blood sugar and weight as this would tell you the risk of diseases linked to your metabolism. Waist circumference in relation to the rest of your body is another indicator of good/bad health and your risk of early death. Last year, an expert group published a paper arguing in particular for waist circumference to be routinely measured by doctors in addition to BMI. Their point is that girth is a vital sign of whether a patient may develop conditions such as type 2 diabetes and heart disease and reducing the width of your middle through diet and exercise should be a priority.

Weighing in

Usually, the only time you discover your BMI is on a trip to the GP. The question is: how and what should you measure yourself at home? For the average person, hopping on the bathroom scales is the traditional way of checking if your weight is going up or down. The three core elements I focused on were:

- daily weight
- blood sugar level
- blood pressure

In the early months of my downsizing, these were the touchstones by which I assessed my progress. You need to start with the basics by dusting off those scales under the bathroom sink or investing in a new (digital) set. Weighing myself wasn't something I did as a kid – only at the doctor's surgery – largely because the not-very-good mechanical scales were basically inaccurate. You'd stand on them, the dial would spin and then come to rest on a number that was usually out by 3lb (1.4kg) either way. In later life, I'd resort to surreptitious checks when staying with friends, but for the most part I avoided bathroom scales because I was scared of bad news and in deep denial. Lying to myself about how heavy I was ended up being a habit I developed over years and found hard to break.

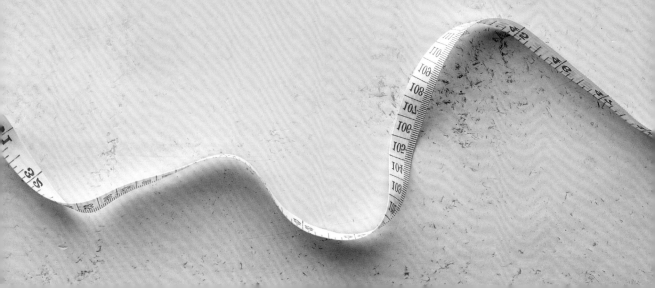

So, committing to buying a pair of scales represented yet another milestone for me. I was finally facing up to the unvarnished reality of my weight. The day I ventured out to buy them is embedded in my memory. The very process of deciding what to go for triggered feelings both of anxiety and excitement. I was about to be awakened from blissful ignorance and to have the awful truth revealed. As a computer game nerd, seeing the data was important for me, so the first set I had the courage to purchase in around 25 years were digital. By linking up the scales to my phone, I could plot the data in MyFitnessPal every day, which in turn produces a graph. To see the graph going down (or up) made me feel more in control of my life.

Let me give you a few tips here from my own experience. Check the maximum weight the scales go up to, because with some I tried I was literally 'off the scale'. The first pair I bought also turned out to be overcomplicated – connecting the scales to my phone took time and a lot of fiddling around. The result was I traded them in for another pair, which were cheaper. Anyone who has bought a modern TV and spent hours trying to make it work will know that simple is sometimes best. Being aware of this and your technical ability (and tolerance threshold) is important, as is checking that the scales are compatible with your phone. Otherwise, it can become another hurdle, an excuse for abandoning your daily measuring.

That said, if you're a scales nerd and enjoy the challenge of technology, then why not invest in a pair that can measure your body fat percentage, body water percentage and muscle mass? Those with smart technology use bio-electrical impedance analysis (BIA) – you place each foot on a pad on the scales which sends a weak electric current through your body and calculates the rate of travel. Body fat causes greater resistance than fat-free zones and therefore slows the speed of the electric current. Just a note of caution: if you've got a pacemaker or are pregnant, then these scales aren't recommended.

When I got home and unboxed my purchase, I stood completely naked in the bathroom of my flat on the new scales. It was August 2017 and not long after my kitchen cupboard detox. The all-important number – 22 stone (140kg) – that registered on the screen was partly shocking and partly to be expected. The positive take from this was I feared I was even heavier, and the negative was that my worst fears had been confirmed. I was morbidly obese.

That was the point, the moment, when I realised I had to commit to preventing my own early death, and to becoming the father who took his children swimming instead of the one who shirked such outings because I was ashamed of wearing trunks in public. But what was the plan of action exactly? In my head I wanted to lose 2lb (0.9kg) in that first week because I'd read this was a reasonable target to hit, although of course the inner (driven) Tom hoped to shed more than this. The notion of anything more daunting, like setting myself a 15-stone (95kg) goal or even getting below 20 stone (127kg), wasn't even on the agenda. I just needed to stop the number on the scales from going up further.

Don't sweat over a few extra pounds

My routine was to weigh myself every morning to keep on track. It had to be morning because I needed to set myself up for the day and to check my weight at a regular time. Evenings were out because of my job, which meant I never knew when I'd be home.

And if the scales showed I'd only lost a pound or two each day, then I didn't freak out. The readings could swing between 3 and 4lb (1.4–1.8kg) either way so I learned not to panic if one day I was heavier than another. At first it was alarming to see my weight seemingly creep up, but the key is to learn that what's important is the overall week-on-week trend. Your water retention is also higher when you're significantly overweight, which is why the weight appears to drop off quicker at the beginning, then slows as the weeks progress.

Here's what my weight looked like the first week of a strict ketogenic eating plan according to the data inputted into MyFitnessPal:

Monday: 281.8lb (127.8kg)

Tuesday: 279.1lb (126.6kg)

Wednesday: 278.9lb (126.5kg)

Thursday: 276.2lb (125.3kg)

Friday: 277.4lb (125.8kg)

Saturday: 274.6lb (124.5kg)

Sunday: 274.8lb (124.6kg)

Total weight loss = 7lb (half a stone) or 3kg

There's a lot of debate around the practice of weighing yourself. Eating disorder charities argue that getting on the scales each day leads to controlling and obsessive behaviour around limiting food intake, a habit that can start in the teenage years. Friends and loved ones who may have anxieties around their own weight may push back too. Some people are unable even to have scales in their home for fear this may trigger negative thoughts and affect their mental health. I absolutely understand where they are coming from, but for me, the act of measuring myself in the morning keeps me aware, throughout the day, of the need to control what I'm putting into my body and how much. It also provides the motivation to be more active, to do my daily steps and to embed a habit. The daily routine made me accountable for my actions – I knew that the bad stuff I ate late at night would appear in the form of a few more pounds on the scales the next day – so it always led to me questioning myself before I reached for foods that were my downfall.

Choosing your scales

I've owned all three of these brands. Withings and Renpho are the two digital ones that provide data I can read on my phone. By far the easiest to set up and connect was the Renpho. It was also cheaper:

Basic
Salter

Better
Withings

Best
Renpho

But if taking charge of your weight isn't for you, then this book probably isn't either. You need to be committed to a lifestyle change and everything that goes with that. By the time I plucked up the courage to stand on the scales, I knew I was nearer to my grave than I should or wanted to be. Being faced with the truth was both shocking and, in a sense, life-affirming – it gave me the wake-up call I desperately needed.

At the start of my downsizing, the weighing routine went like this. First, I'd get out of bed and go to the toilet (in the hope I'd weigh less!), then walk into the kitchen, put the kettle on and weigh myself. While the kettle was boiling, I'd test my blood sugar levels. Although I could digitally monitor my weight, there was no way of being able to capture my blood sugar. What I did was keep a small notepad by the kettle where I'd systematically write the date, my weight and my blood sugar levels (see page 72 for details on how to measure blood sugar). At the end of the week, I'd go back through the numbers and see how well I was progressing.

This all sounds quite hardcore but it's important in the early stages because you turn it into a habit. Once it becomes a habit, then the whole routine probably takes around 3–5 minutes max a day. And it becomes a normal part of your daily life.

Food logging: how to measure your food intake

The next measurement for the rest of the day was how many calories I was consuming and their nutritional content. Known as food logging, there are plenty of programmes and free or paid-for apps out there to make the whole process easier. You just need to find one that works for you and put aside some time to set them up. Most people go straight to MyFitnessPal – of all the apps I paid for, I know I'll be using this for the rest of my life. Compatible with Apple's iPhone, the app also works with Android devices. MyFitnessPal isn't perfect (nothing is) but it works because you can log your weight and scan barcodes, which gives instant nutrient levels for all the foods you need. The data revolution has meant it is now easy to see how horrific the sugar content is in foods. I'd scan a can of fizzy drink, then hastily delete it from my log.

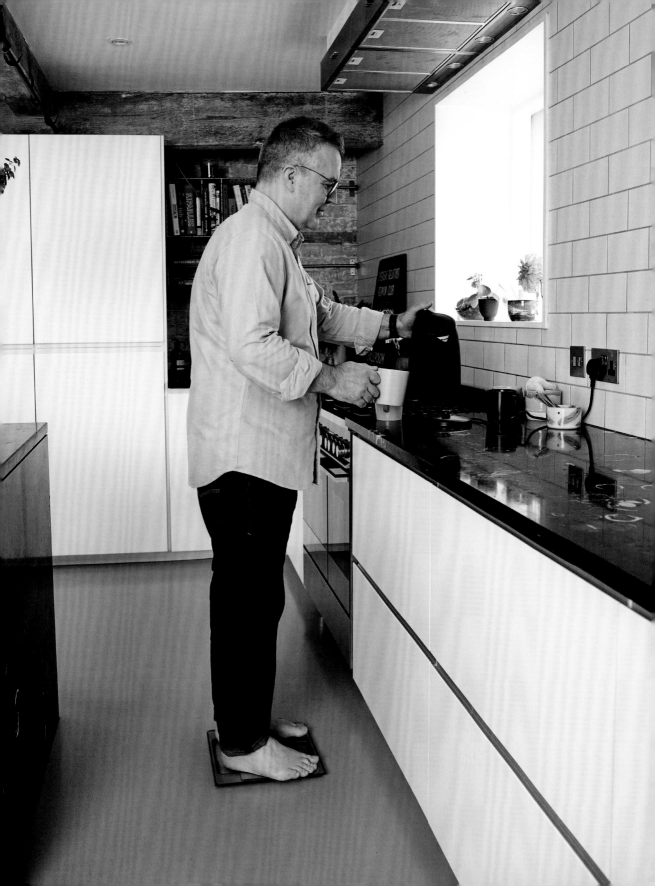

And the app remembers what you've eaten in previous meals, making it simple to add this information to your food log. The app creates a pie chart of the percentage of each macronutrient you've consumed as well as the calorific value. So over time you build up a valuable store of data, even down to how much vitamin C you're consuming. The app also allows you to log the time you eat, which means you can tell if you're falling into bad habits such as eating late at night, too close to going to bed.

Like weighing yourself on the scales, some people will tell you not to measure what you eat, but as I was on a strict Keto diet, where the allowance of carbs is 20g or less a day, I found it very useful. A breakfast was usually a standard plate of eggs and bacon. With the app, I felt more in control and had a sense of where I was on my weight-loss journey. At first, I was quite obsessive about monitoring my food intake but now, four years on, I'm more relaxed about it and know I can return to food logging if bad habits are creeping in.

Keeping a check on your grazing

Make sure you enter the details of all the food you eat – the stuff you graze on counts too and can often be the root of excessive weight gain. It's that sense of 'It doesn't really count' that can be your downfall. It certainly has been mine, especially as the foods you eat outside of meals often contain hidden calories like those coffees laced with syrup. Or the block of cheese you've casually munched through while looking for something 'healthy' in the fridge. To combat cravings, what I'd often do when out would be to buy a piece of lean, protein-packed chicken and go and sit in a coffee shop. You're exercising personal choice and choosing a snack that isn't packed with thousands of calories.

You may be thinking how you go about food logging when you're with friends or work contacts? Don't be put off logging by thinking you'll feel silly. Everyone was incredibly generous when I told them what I needed to do. I'd tell them at the start of the meal/lunch meeting that I was on a 'crazy' diet and did they mind if I just took a few seconds (because that's all it takes) to log what I was eating.

Getting over the embarrassment factor and being disciplined is crucial. After all, what's more important: your health or what others think? From flexitarian to pescatarian, so many people now have different approaches to eating anyway that you'll find you're not alone and may even find it's an ice-breaker.

My first ever food log

Believe it or not, this was what I used to consider a healthy-ish day of eating:

Breakfast – 2 large eggs, 1 avocado, 2 slices of wholemeal bread, large cafétiere of coffee

Lunch (bistro meal) – crab salad, spaghetti carbonara, mixed salad

Dinner – breaded chicken breast and 2 rollmop herrings

Drinks (not including tea and water) – 4 glasses of rosé and 1 glass white wine spritzer

Total intake: 2,348 calories, 43% fat, 33% carbohydrate, 24% protein

What are macronutrients?

Many eating plans focus on the amount of protein, fat and carbohydrate in your diet. They are the three essential elements that your body needs in large amounts for energy. Hence the term, 'macro' nutrient. Food logging allows you to work out the ratio between the three if you're trying (as I was) to keep carb levels down.

Fat 1g = 9 calories

Protein 1g = 4 calories

Carbohydrate 1g = 4 calories

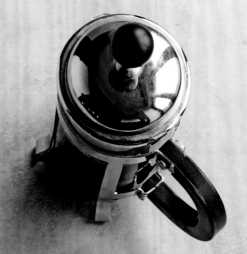

Tracking your steps

Some people swear by pedometers, Fitbits or Apple watches, which will do all the basics for you in tracking how much and how far you move on a daily basis. My lifestyle meant I was practically glued to my phone all day, so I just used the steps count on it. Not everyone has the freedom to access their phone all day, though. If this is the case, a step tracker can be useful – my view is they're not particularly accurate but that's not necessarily important. The key thing is you are setting yourself a baseline measurement that allows you to monitor your activity.

MyFitnessPal will take the data from your phone and work out your weekly, monthly and annual steps average. You end up with a picture over time of what your general activity levels are, and by that I mean when you're not actually exercising but *moving*. When I was actively losing weight at the start of my journey, I would closely monitor how many steps I was doing daily. The correlation between what I achieved and my efforts to fight the flab was striking.

Controlling blood pressure

To add to all my health woes, my blood pressure was *severely* high at one stage, which required treatment with medication. Hypertension (high blood pressure) happens to be common in my family, a fact I seized upon to delude myself that my condition was totally down to genes and nothing to do with my food-addicted, exercise-poor lifestyle. Checking my blood pressure each day became an essential part of my measuring routine once I finally faced up to the fact that I could actually do something about my health. The readings were both a source of anxiety and a source of motivation to get my exercise kit on, get out of the door and get active.

The dangers of high blood pressure

When you get a blood pressure reading there will be two numbers. The higher number is the force (systolic pressure) at which blood is pumped around your body by the heart. The lower one (diastolic) is how much resistance there is in your blood vessels to this blood flow. An estimated 1 in 3 adults in the UK have high blood pressure (according to the NHS, this is if it is more than 140/90) but many don't have obvious symptoms such as headaches, dizziness and shortness of breath. They only discover they have the condition when they get their reading checked. Left untreated, the disease increases your risk of serious problems such as heart attacks and strokes by putting extra strain on your blood vessels. What can occur is these vessels become weakened inside the brain, then bleed on and into surrounding tissues. The blood accumulates, puts pressure on brain tissue and triggers damage.

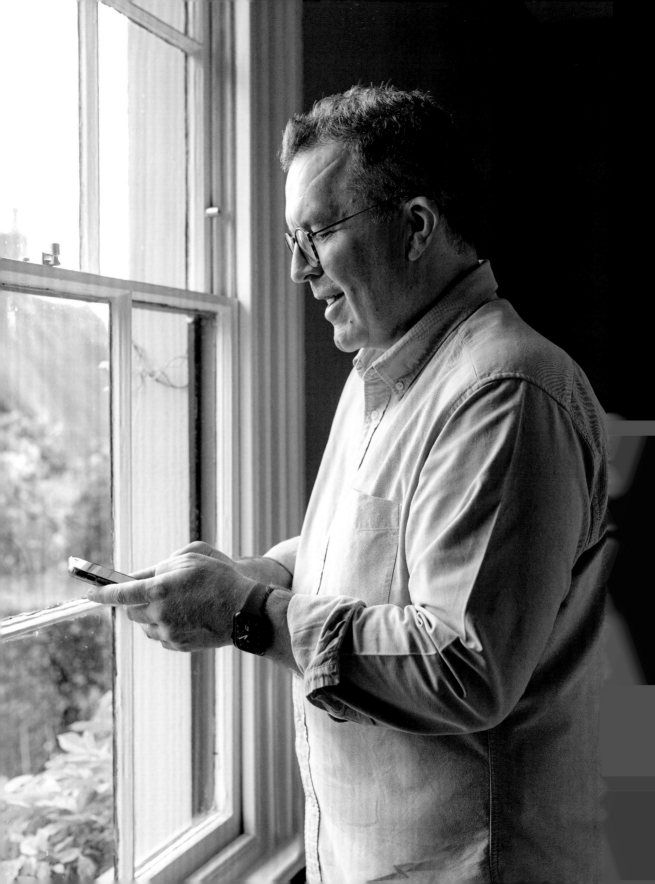

Counting ketones

This only applies if you're following a ketogenic diet (see page 52), which I did in the early stages of my downsizing. My mission was to reach a state of ketosis where my body was drawing down energy from fat stores. What I needed to establish was whether I'd reached the level necessary to trigger fat-burning in order to reduce my excessive weight and tackle my insulin resistance. Another finger-prick test was required to check if my ketone levels had reached the optimum measurement of 1.5–3.0 mmol/l. Using a monitor, I'd check the figure, and combine it with my blood glucose reading to come up with a ratio that would indicate if I had achieved the desired goal. This is often called the Glucose Ketone Index (GKI). It's not essential to get to this level of detail but I found it helpful, and if I could spend most of my time in a moderate level of ketosis I was happy. As well as always contributing to weight loss, I also felt more mentally sharp, like my brain fog had lifted.

Glucose Ketone Index (GKI)	Reading	Application
9 or above	Not in ketosis	
6–9	Low level of ketosis	For weight loss or health maintenance.
3–6	Moderate level of ketosis	For managing type 2 diabetes and obesity, insulin resistance, metabolic or endocrine disorders.
1–3	High therapeutic level of ketosis	For those using keto therapeutically for the treatment of diseases such as cancer, epilepsy, Alzheimer's, Parkinson's, traumatic brain injury, etc.
less than 1	The highest therapeutic level of ketosis	Very difficult to achieve and shouldn't be reached without a doctor's supervision.

- Following a one-size-fits-all approach to food isn't necessarily best, so create your own tailored downsizing eating programme.

- Healthy blood pressure, blood sugar levels, waist circumference and cholesterol (HDL) adds up to good metabolic health, and this means less risk of dying early from diseases such as diabetes and stroke.

- Consider investing in a continuous glucose monitor that provides you with readings day and night to combat fluctuating blood sugar levels that can throw your body into turmoil and will reduce your chance of weight loss.

- Weighing yourself, checking blood sugar levels and blood pressure and food logging should be part of your daily routine in your early days of downsizing.

- An app such as MyFitnessPal can help you record the calorie/nutritional content of every meal – make sure you include any grazing.

- MyFitnessPal is also an easy way to track your steps by taking data from your phone to work out your weekly, monthly and annual steps to build up a picture over time of activity levels.

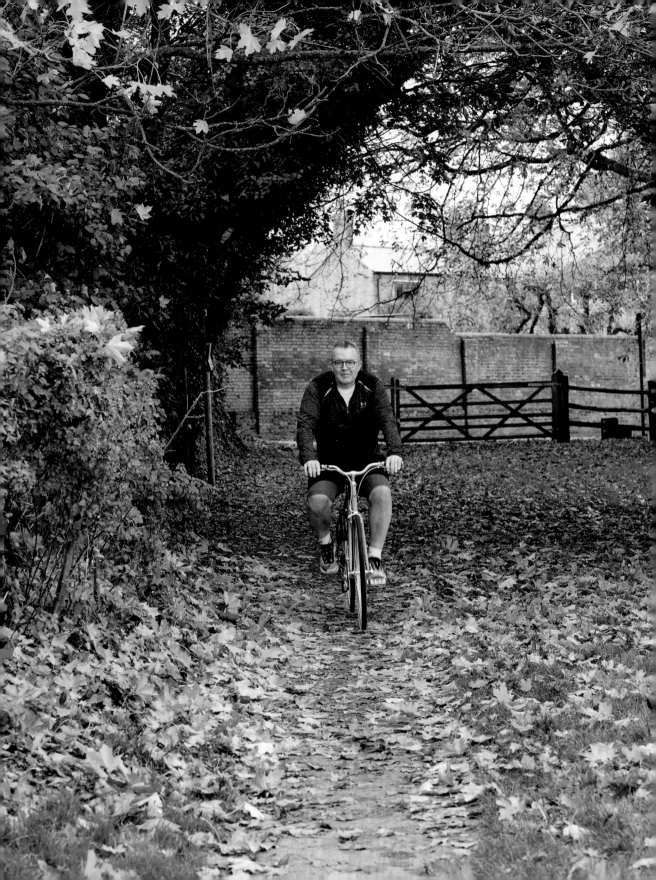

4 Movement

Exercise may be a way of getting the calories out of you. It's not a way of stopping them coming in, especially the empty ones that provide the body with no benefits and in fact pose a danger to health. That said, any weight-loss plan usually involves some increased physical activity. It's not particularly scientific but I would say that the success ratio is probably 80 per cent nutrition and 20 per cent exercise. The calories you consume need to be burned off through activity, and you can't be active without having sufficient energy in the form of food to make your muscles function properly. This is especially true if, like me, you want to reverse type 2 diabetes.

Getting out of the starting blocks

The first thought after 'I must lose weight' is 'I must exercise more'. That's when sweaty panic sets in, even hard-to-suppress feelings of wanting to vomit. For most people, exercise means pounding the streets from dawn to dusk, signing up for the first marathon they find on Facebook or being barked at by a personal trainer who resembles a still-feared teacher from their school days.

Stop right there. Just slow down, breathe deeply and take a moment before you even begin to contemplate spending lots of money you may not have on a fancy bike. Or rush into an endurance challenge that will end with you crumpled in a sweaty heap way before the finish line. Exercise is important for a long and healthy life but it's not the *only* solution.

When embarking on a weight-loss programme, the trap so many of us fall into is to use a cycle ride, run or swim as an excuse for eating more calories instead of properly addressing diet and nutrition. Who hasn't left a training session feeling virtuous and thought 'I've earned that chocolate bar/bag of crisps/glass of wine'?

As a teen I played a lot of sport but became less active once I began work – and that's when the weight piled on. Dr Michael Mosley has written about how inactivity is often the root cause of insulin resistance. This is a condition where the body's cells no longer react as they should to the hormone insulin. What happens is these cells start to ignore the signals from the pancreas to tell them to take up glucose from the bloodstream. The result is the pancreas overcompensates by producing more and more insulin. Over time, the organ gets worn out and sugar levels in the blood can rise. And that can lead to type 2 diabetes.

If you're not moving your muscles much, fat, Mosley says, accumulates in them gradually, and this leads to the development of insulin resistance. And I know from experience that this silent disease can take you to a very unhealthy place. The flip side of this is that the more you move, the greater your chance of reversing type 2 diabetes. Desperation and hopelessness don't have to be your future if you take control now and build activity into your daily life. The body can recover by using insulin effectively once again, which in turn results in stabilised glucose levels in the blood.

Breaking out of a sedentary regime isn't easy. Especially if you have the added challenge of being seriously overweight, as I was. But there are ways of boosting activity levels without resorting to an extreme fitness plan. The secret is to keep it simple instead of believing the only way is to shell out money for a gym membership that you may never even use again after the first trip. What's also key is making a conscious effort to sit down with your diary and allocate time for exercise in your busy schedule. I give you tips about this on page 94. These are not radical suggestions that will require you to leave everything (and everyone) you know

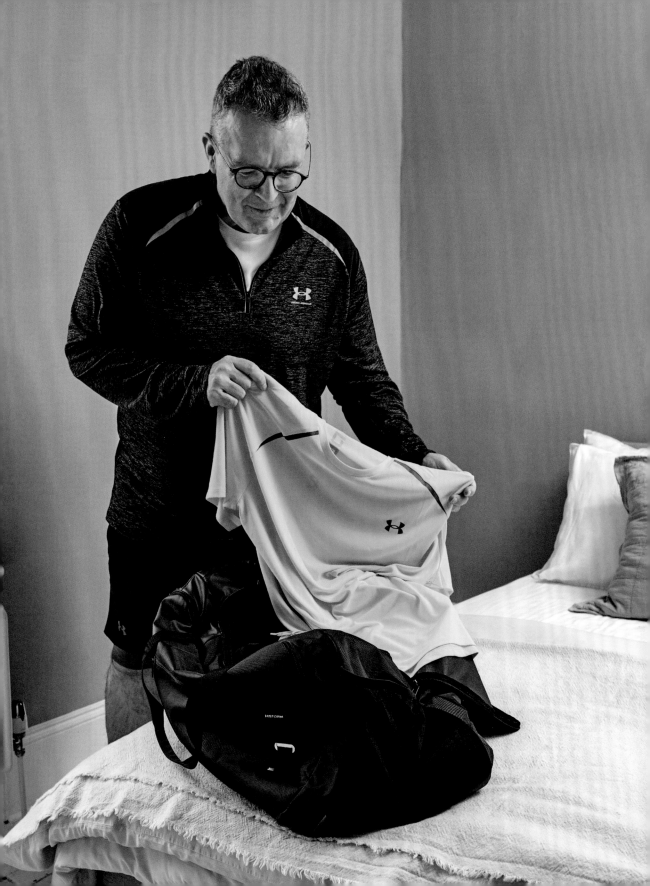

and love behind. I'm not suggesting you resign immediately from your office job, stop the computer games or ditch watching TV (or even get rid of the television set altogether). What I am recommending – and what worked for me – is making physical activity (especially walking) part of your daily routine along with getting up from your chair/sofa as often as you can.

Activity for life

The first step to moving more is not spending so many hours a day sitting down. Obvious, I know, but this is the unhealthy reality for millions of workers who do jobs that involve working at a desk. All the evidence suggests that sitting down for extended periods without getting up every half hour to stretch your legs can seriously harm your health (see box on page 94). And I was part of this chained-to-your-desk and long working hours culture for the best part of three decades. A trend that has persisted – even increased – as a result of the pandemic with more people doing their jobs from home. An international study that looked at the impact on eating and physical activity of being confined at home during COVID-19 found that daily sitting time alone increased from 5 to 8 hours a day. The intensity levels of physical activity that people achieved also declined, and they took to snacking between meals more. I'm sure the latter was down to the temptation of being within easy reach of the fridge and all the calorific delights within.

If you are spending too long on your bottom and not on your feet because you're stuck in front of your laptop, then there are ways to get active, or if you fit the couch potato category of being glued to the TV, this is what you can do to kick-start your metabolism, get your muscles working and reduce your risk of serious health problems:

- Stand up from your chair (or sofa) at least once an hour and shake out your feet and hands.

- Try suggesting 'walking' meetings to your work colleagues.

- Start the day with a 10-minute brisk walk.

Another tip is to try a standing desk – basically one that allows you to work comfortably while on your feet. Just compare the difference in calories burned between standing and sitting. To keep your body upright, your body uses muscles and that requires fuel for them to function. In 1 hour, standing adds up to approximately 206 calories burned for the average 12 stone (77kg) person vs 134 calories if you're sitting down.

Some studies say that even those who do light exercise can still cut their risk of death from heart problems. The Copenhagen City Heart Study followed 5,000 people over five years and split them into two groups. They found that those who did light-moderate jogging had the lowest risk of death, compared to the joggers who pounded the pavement breaking a sweat.

> Swapping a 12-minute stroll for a 7-minute brisk walk reduces your risk of early death.

In fact, the strenuous joggers had the same mortality rate as sedentary people who did nothing.

And time isn't necessarily of the essence when it comes to how long you spend exercising in a single session. A Cambridge University study concluded that you can reduce your risk of death simply by swapping a 12-minute stroll for a 7-minute brisk walk. This was after looking at data from 90,000 people wearing fitness trackers over two years. So, if you've fewer minutes to spare it doesn't have to be a barrier.

Say no to sedentary and get walking!

A sedentary lifestyle – one with a lot of sitting/lying down and little exercise – is the curse of the modern age. The minimum recommended levels for movement are at least 150 minutes a week of moderate-intensity physical activity. That's the recommendation for adults from The World Health Organization. Following this target can bring numerous health benefits, including a reduced risk of type 2 diabetes, cardiovascular disease and some cancers.

Yet according to *The Miracle Pill* by writer Peter Walker, 2 in 5 British adults are so inactive they don't meet these recommendations. Walker quotes data from Public Health England showing that over 6.3 million adults aged 40 to 60 don't achieve 10 minutes of continuous brisk walking over the course of a month. What's even more worrying is that we Brits walk 15 miles less a year than we did two decades ago.

In her book *Move!*, the science writer Caroline Williams reveals that the average person now spends 70% of their time sitting or lying around – and that was before the pandemic forced many of us to retreat indoors for weeks at a time. Williams highlights the deadly effects of inactivity using a celebrated research study from the 1950s. The author of the research, British epidemiologist Dr Jeremy N Morris, was the first person to analyse the link between cardiovascular disease and lack of movement. Morris looked at workers who spent their day driving double-decker buses in London. What he found was that they were twice as likely to

What a sedentary lifestyle does to your body

Any calories your body doesn't need are converted into a type of fat called triglycerides. So, the less active you are, the higher the triglyceride levels circulating in your blood. Imagine all that fat just floating around in your arteries, especially if you're spending hours a day at a desk hardly moving. If you're sitting down for more than 20 minutes, your body puts the process of removing this fat from your body on hold. High triglyceride levels are a factor in artery walls thickening. Clogged arteries increase the risk of stroke, heart attack and heart disease, but exercise increases the levels in your blood of 'good' (HDL) cholesterol, which can lower triglyceride levels. Just getting up every 20 minutes will have a dramatic and positive impact.

die of heart disease as those who were employed as bus conductors, the people selling tickets and collecting fares. While the drivers spent the day sitting down at the wheel, the conductors moved around the bus. Of course, they weren't running marathons or doing punishing exercise – the ticket collectors weren't even getting out of breath unless chasing a fare dodger. What they were doing was going up and down the stairs regularly. So as a result they suffered far less heart disease purely because they had regular (if slow) movement around the bus.

The take-home message from this is that movement – any movement – is a good place to start, rather than thinking you have to take up extreme sports from day one of your weight-loss journey. If you're in the 1 in 5 of the population who has type 2 diabetes, as I was, don't think you're a hopeless case beyond help. Before downsizing, I was definitely in the 'couch potato' category – a 10-minute walk was not something I valued or felt

I needed to make time for. Instead, my bad habit was a short black-cab ride between meetings in Whitehall and Westminster. Sometimes, I would travel just half a mile for the minimum fare of £5. Not only did this hit me in the pocket, it was undermining my health and wellbeing.

If you've entered middle age (or are well into it like me), there's the added whammy of the natural ageing process which brings with it hard-to-shift fat around the waist known as the 'spare tyre'. Yet just a little bit of movement on a daily basis can make all the difference. The evidence shows that at least one brisk 10-minute daily walk reduces the risk of early death by 15%. Yes, just devoting a few minutes a day to a limited amount of movement can reap rewards, which is good news for the 2 in 5 people who find it hard to get off the sofa, including those who are diabetic.

How can you achieve this if you've got a hectic lifestyle? Breaking down challenges into easy-to-achieve habits is an effective strategy, as I outlined on page 28. So, to achieve

> The less active we
> are the less well
> our brains work.

150 minutes of activity a week, think of it as two sessions lasting 10 minutes every day with an extra 10 minutes at the weekend. That doesn't sound so bad, or too difficult to achieve, does it?

To make things even easier, there are apps available that show when you're walking briskly. The Active 10 tracker developed by the NHS is free to use and just needs to be kept in a pocket close to your body to measure your activity levels. Downloaded onto a smartphone, the app also tells you when to increase the pace and how to fit more walking into your day.

Walking is the antidote to a sedentary lifestyle. It was the strategy I adopted as part of my weight-loss programme and by the end I was covering 4–5 miles a day walking around central London without giving it a second thought. There were even social benefits – sometimes my colleagues and I would walk around Westminster at lunchtime, including down to the National Theatre and Royal Festival Hall. When it rained, then we would just walk up and down the corridors of the House of Commons. Lots of strange things go on in politics, so the sight of us walking up and down didn't attract too many stares.

Your mind health, focus and creative thinking powers will also improve through walking. In his book In *Praise of Walking*, neuroscientist Shane O'Mara writes about not only the physical but also the mental and physiological impact of movement. He argues that movement is essentially a superpower – it boosts our wellbeing as well as making us healthier, and also unlocks the brain's cognitive powers. O'Mara supports a view that the brain is 'motor-centric', which means it has evolved to support movement. Our sensory systems (for example, sight and touch) are stimulated the more we're out and about experiencing the world instead of sat at a desk. But if we stop that activity, the grey matter will cease to work as well as before.

There are a host of other experts who are cheerleaders for working your legs and feet. Professor Vybarr Cregan-Reid from the University of Kent even goes as far to describe walking as a 'miracle cure'. His book, *Primate Change*, documents how we've gone from walking through ancient grasslands to hardly using our feet at all and explains that this is doing irreparable harm to our bodies. We're suffering because of our lifestyles, and technology is largely to blame. Constantly checking Facebook, updating your Instagram feed or sending endless WhatsApp messages might be considered by many to be essential to happiness, but being outdoors and moving our bodies provides a dopamine boost that actually does us good and increases our chances of living longer.

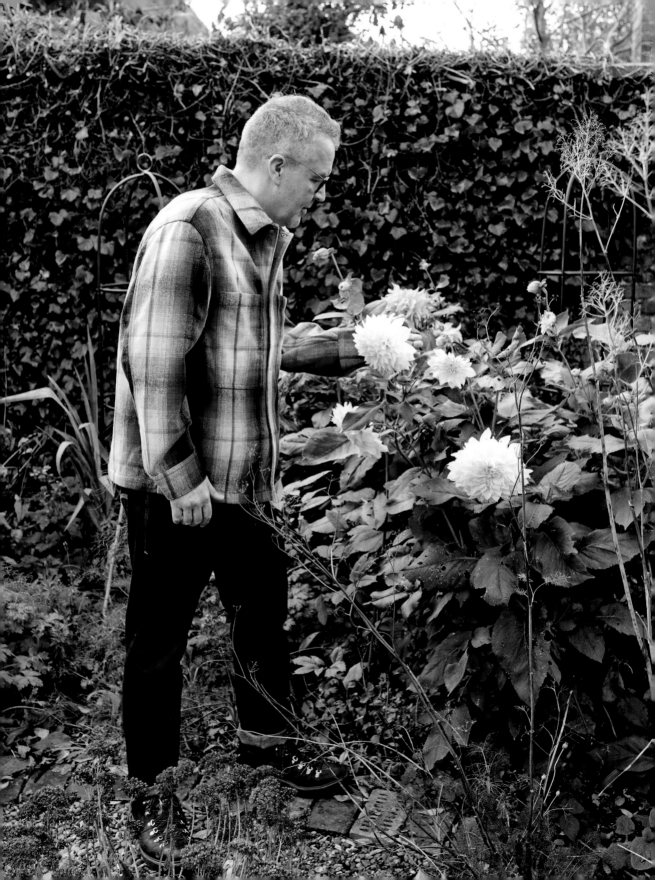

Giving your heart a boost

The number one role of the heart is to pump oxygen-rich blood around the body to keep organs healthy and functioning properly. Movement and exercise have numerous benefits for the heart, including improved blood flow. Better circulation in the small vessels around the organ is one such bonus – this may even prevent heart attacks by ensuring blood moves normally all around the body. When your heart's pumping efficiently, it's helping to reduce cholesterol, which is linked to cardiovascular disease. Some studies have shown that exercise can increase the movement of bad fats (LDL) out of the blood into the liver and from there out of the body altogether. Other evidence suggests that being active leads to other improvements related to cholesterol, such as increasing levels of good (HDL) fats. The more you work your body and your heart, the better your heart performs under stress and the quicker it recovers after exercise. What happens is that your body becomes trained to move oxygen from the blood to muscles, which need it to function.

Regular movement and physical activity also strengthen the heart muscle, which means it needs less effort to pump blood and can circulate more of the red stuff around the body. When your heart is healthy, it pushes out more blood with every beat instead of being sluggish. The overall upside is lower blood pressure – there's less force needed to push blood through your arteries. And if blood pressure is reduced again, you have less chance of a heart attack, stroke and even vascular dementia.

What is moderate intensity exercise?

The answer is anything that gets your heart rate up to 50% or higher than the rate when resting. It's not as fast as you would imagine and can be achieved by:

- Brisk walking
- Riding a bike
- Pushing a lawnmower
- Dancing
- Gardening
- Climbing stairs

Step forward

The antidote to a sedentary lifestyle is walking and at the core of this activity is a daily steps target. Aiming for 5,000 steps a day is a good start – it's what I did at the beginning of my journey, and If I could achieve this, then so can you, every day for as long as you are able.

To many, steps don't mean a lot. To put this measurement into context, 5,000 steps are the equivalent of around 2.5 miles or 4km. The thought of that much exertion would have filled me with dread a few years ago and seemed the equivalent of climbing Mount Snowdon. Fast forward to 2019 and I actually *did* climb that Welsh peak (the highest in Wales), thanks to keeping to my daily steps routine combined with my exercise and healthy eating programme. This was one of many physical fitness challenges that I would never have thought possible before.

For the rest of your life you will be walking more, and you have to accept this fact. If you're going to lose weight and maintain it, then there's no end goal as such – putting one foot in front of the other in a meaningful way has to be what you do forever. The good news is that it's safe, has low impact on your body and joints, and is simple to do. Walking doesn't have to mean striding outdoors in a howling gale in sub-zero temperatures like an Arctic explorer. Steps can be incorporated into your life in so many other ways, such as putting the bins out, doing DIY or cleaning the car, and some don't even involve leaving your house, for example moving around your office, walking upstairs and jogging on the spot.

Before you start

Setting a weekly steps target will help reset your life. A few days before the start of your weight-loss plan, get monitoring how many steps you are actually doing by using a pedometer or a fitness app. The initial aim should be 5,000, which is the threshold for an active lifestyle and defined as 'low active'. Imagine burning off 100 calories a day by walking alone. That's roughly what you'd lose in 5,000 steps depending on your height/weight/speed, and the equivalent of over 360,000 calories in a decade.

If you're already doing more than this, great. Add another 10% to your current total. If you're not at this point, then don't worry – set your sights on 5,000. Over the years I've increased my target to 10,000 (the equivalent of around five miles or 8km) and I never go below this, unless I'm going through a setback, which means I need to do a reset.

The real danger point to health is fewer than 5,000 steps a day. Researchers that have investigated the issue of activity and health have established that people whose activity levels are not high enough to reach 5,000 steps have sedentary lifestyles. As I've already detailed, lack of activity is associated with a range of diseases, including diabetes.

Walking can boost your imagination and lead to 'light-bulb' moments

Billions of nerve cells pack our brain and these generate electricity (albeit in tiny amounts) in the form of brainwaves. The four categories of brainwaves include theta, which are associated with learning, memory and daydreaming. According to Professor O'Mara, theta can be detected during movement. You may have noticed that conversation flows more easily and is more inspired when you go for a walk with someone (your partner, for example). Or the solution to a problem floats into your mind without having to force it or overthink. O'Mara points out that great thinkers and philosophers through the ages have used the inspirational power of walking. The celebrated polymath Bertrand Russell credited a stroll with being integral to his work and would walk for an hour every morning in order to be motivated to write for the rest of the day. Other walking enthusiasts include Charles Darwin. The author of *On the Origin of Species* even created his own 'thinking path' in the grounds of his home Down House, in Kent, where he strolled morning and afternoon while working on his famous theory of evolution.

A study published in the journal *Sports Medicine* looked into the use of pedometers and recommendations for how many steps a day are enough to maintain good health.

Their conclusions were:

- 5,000 to 7,499 steps a day = 'low active'

- 7,500 to 9,999 steps a day = 'somewhat active'

- 10,000 to 12,499 a day = 'active'

- More than 12,500 steps a day = 'highly active'

Take time to think about/plan how you're going to achieve your daily steps goal. If you don't prepare, then you risk being stalled by inventing excuses for yourself, such as *'I need to order sports socks'* or *'I can't find any trainers that fit'*. The good news is that you don't need to buy fancy kit to get active. If you're planning to trek long distances over rugged terrain, then of course invest in a pair of walking boots that fit properly and protect you from painful blisters. But for short trips, a pair of comfortable trainers to support your feet will do.

The Science of Steps

The concept of 'steps' is believed to have originated in Japan in the 1960s. The country was hosting the 1964 Olympics, which triggered awareness about the need to get fit. This coincided with the introduction of pedometers too, and a walking craze – called Manpo-Kei (meaning 10,000 steps) – took off. Walking clubs sprang up dedicated to 10,000 steps as a minimum target and eventually it became a trend that was adopted around the world and endures to this day. In 2005, a study undertaken by Ghent University in Belgium in collaboration with the University of Queensland in Australia investigated whether 10,000 steps a day benefitted those who achieved this target. The researchers studied those encouraged to reach this target through a community-based programme and found an 8% increase in the number of people reaching 10,000 steps by the end of a year. This compared with no increase among those not taking part in the programme. The average daily increase for those taking part in the study was 896, though a follow-up found the effect wasn't maintained after four years, by which point the average was around 100 steps higher and overall the number of steps reverted to the amount taken at the start of the trial. Physical activity in the intervention group, however, didn't decrease. The thinking now among experts is that 10,000 steps isn't necessarily a magic number. More recent research by Dr I-Min Lee published in 2019 found that even those doing fewer than 10,000 steps a day (8,000) are half as likely to die early from heart disease or other causes than those doing 4,000 steps. And the good news appears to be that even those who manage fewer than 5,000 steps a day (4,400) can reduce their risk of premature death by 40% compared with those doing 2,700 or fewer. The key message is that even movement below the golden figure of 5 miles a day can preserve our longevity.

Next steps

After establishing space in your day to walk at least 5,000 steps, if you're comfortable with this activity and find it easy, you can add a few more rules to your daily routine. Find time to review your walking stats. If you've hit your target, give yourself a silent mental high-five.

Aim to walk up every set of steps you come to (and ditch the lift). Doing this left me gasping for breath at first, but over time it became second nature. Remember – small actions and life adjustments become habits upon which you can build.

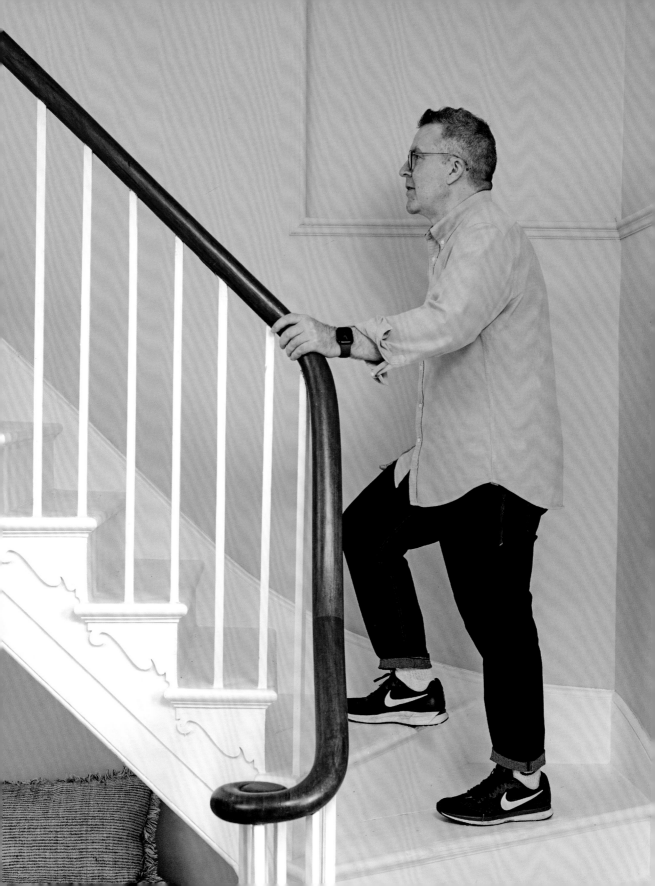

Doing it daily

At the core of getting more active is daily activity, and walking is key to this. If you want to get on your bike and do 10km in one session, that's great. For many, though, this isn't a realistic target or there may be times when it's simply not possible because of time or other constraints. The point I'm making here is don't ever lose sight of walking as your basic regime. The benefits are numerous and include loss of body fat, relief of back pain, improvement in mood and lower blood pressure. That's why it should be your 'currency' for moving every day – other activities can always be 'bolted on' to walking. By the end of my downsizing, I was doing my daily steps, which I'd enhance with other activities such as cycling to the supermarket for my weekly shop instead of taking the car.

For more than a decade, I'd regarded having to walk from my office to the House of Commons to vote as a chore and I resented it. It wasn't taking part in the democratic process that irritated me – I'd given my life to politics and was utterly dedicated to the people I was elected to represent. No, it was the fact that having to walk to the chamber was an unwelcome interruption in my already packed day and the physical effort that came with it. Although my office was relatively close to the chamber, it was up a flight of 60-odd steps. The light-bulb moment came when I embarked on my downsizing journey and my discovery of a steps target. What was once a bothersome task became an ideal opportunity to get in my daily steps, a gift that I now relished.

I've mentioned how you need to get your friends and colleagues on side to support you in your downsizing goals. My team was relatively young and very encouraging in my fitness crusade, so much so that they embraced the idea of attending 'walking' meetings – we'd literally walk down the corridors of the Commons, talking as we went. However, the world of work and has changed significantly since the pandemic, with many employees still meeting virtually. Along with other home-based workers, I found myself spending more time sitting in my office chair then I ever did during my entire 19 years as an MP.

There are ways, though, of combining work with movement. Get up off your chair, stand up while interacting on Zoom, walk from room to room while talking on the phone. You could also set a reminder on your phone to make sure you move every hour, and set weekly steps goals with colleagues. In the previous chapter on Measurement, I explained how to track your steps to give a picture of how much you're doing (see page 84). I promise if you get your monthly average steps up it will have a significant impact on your life and downsizing goal.

The steps to miles equation

2,000 steps = about 1 mile

5,000 steps = 2.2 miles (slow walk) or 3 miles (run)

Calories burned =100–300

Climbing 20 steps burns 15 calories on the way up and 5 on the way down.

Steps case study

For my ITV documentary *Giving Up Sugar: For Good?*, I interviewed a range of people about their health and fitness, including Dan, a shift worker in a factory. In his job, he had to do a lot of traipsing around – this was a part of his work role but was activity he resented. Sometimes Dan's daily steps would total 16,000, which is the equivalent of nearly 6 miles if he was walking at a very slow pace or over 8 if he was walking briskly. Over time, he changed his mindset about what he'd previously regarded as a chore. What Dan did was to build the steps into his own bespoke fitness regime and create a target for how many steps he did at work. Walking became a source of enjoyment to such an extent that he would end up getting irritated when not at work because he was not walking as much as he was during the week.

How to measure your steps

There are plenty of apps out there that measure your steps, including the Active 10 app, developed by the NHS, which records every minute of walking you do. Remember the WHO guidelines of 150 minutes exercise a week? That's the equivalent of two 10-minute brisk walks a day with an extra 10 minutes slotted in at the weekend. Many of the early research studies on steps were done with pedometers that are worn around the waist. Now many fitness trackers are worn around the wrist and may count arm movements as steps, which is why they've been criticised for accuracy. What I did was to use the stopwatch on my phone to work out my average per minute (in my case it was 125 paces).

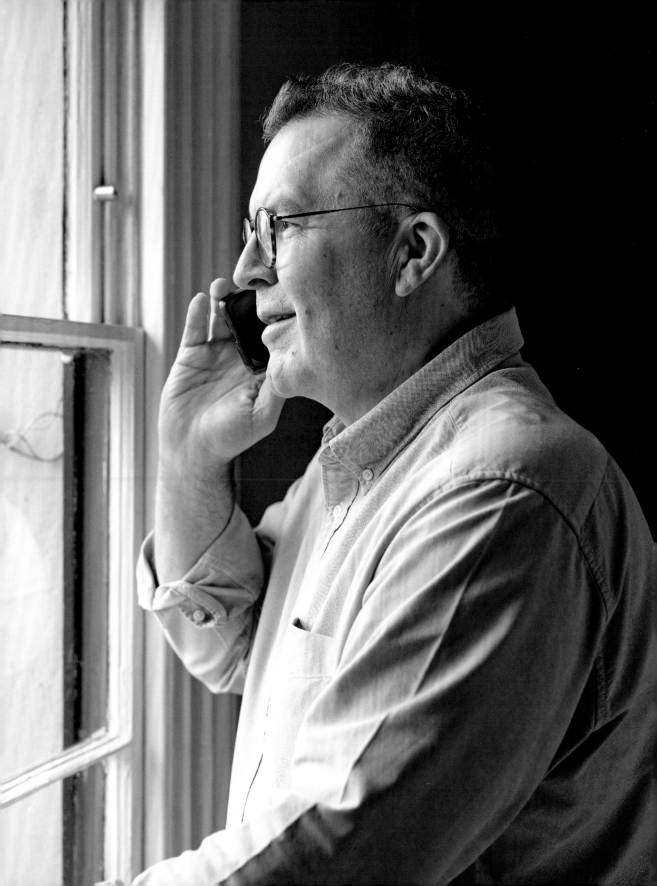

2 minutes marching on the spot can add 240 steps towards your daily target.

Getting steps into your daily routine

I've mentioned ways of reaching your daily steps target when at home or working. There are plenty of other little tricks you can employ when faced with time on your hands that you can't otherwise fill. One of mine was to be creative with the 20 minutes waiting for a train at Birmingham Moor Street station. Instead of standing in one spot or sitting down in the waiting room, I'd spend the time walking up and down the platform, which always attracted glances from the station guards. A 'pace-while-you-wait' approach can also be used while you're waiting in queues, for the kettle to boil, for the bathroom to empty of family members or (once you get in there) brushing your teeth. Just 2 minutes spent marching on the spot can add up to 240 steps towards your daily target.

Getting off your bus or train stop early and walking the extra distance you'd have taken by train can also boost your count. Then there are the trips to the supermarket that may seem like a chore but can be viewed as a chance to work in some steps on the walk from the car park to the store. Even the drag of having to take the trolley back can be turned into an opportunity to move more.

What about holidays? Doing steps while everyone else is determined to relax and exercise is probably the last thing on your mind. Well, the secret is to get your steps in before your family/friends wake up. Not drinking heavily is a plus because it means you're often up before anyone else rather than sleeping off a hangover. On a holiday to Torremolinos in Spain, I was greeted by half a dozen post-booze-session pals who had to do a double take at the sight of me repeatedly pacing around the pool. You're basically ahead of the game if you manage your time effectively and the sense of satisfaction is enormous. And it means you've got the rest of the day to relax or play.

Swapping the washing machine for a laundry mangle is a step too far. That said, cutting out some modern conveniences such as the carwash and doing it by hand instead can boost your activity rate. As I said in the section on mindset (see page 28), it's about changing your internal narrative. What seems an obstacle can be turned into an opportunity and a reward for meeting your goals.

Embarking on exercise

Earlier I said that day one of your downsizing journey is not the right time to sign up to a gym or fitness centre. You probably won't be ready to take this step, are therefore more likely to quit despite all good intentions, be destined for failure and punish yourself as a result. Instead, you need to get your healthy eating schedule sorted and think about the activity targets you want to meet each day. Once you're on track with these, you can think about what exercise you want to do in addition to your daily steps.

When you start to lose weight, you'll reach a point quite soon into your journey where you find yourself with more energy. This is the point at which you might want to apply yourself to physical fitness as well as weight loss. Why is fitness important as part of your downsizing programme? Surely eating healthily, losing weight and hitting your daily steps target is enough? After all, you're already moving the odds of a longer life in the right direction. The simple answer is that getting fitter further reduces the risk of serious illness, especially heart disease.

There's no shortage of activities out there and there's one to suit everyone's abilities and preferences. It may be dancing, Pilates or yoga that gets you hooked, or swimming or tennis. Given I've two left feet and no co-ordination, the exercise regime that worked for me, in addition to my daily steps, was based around cycling and gym-related workouts. Everyone is different though. Be led by what works for you and importantly what suits your lifestyle and pocket. The expert view is that what's key is to incorporate the four pillars of fitness because each has different benefits:

• strength

• aerobic flexibility

• balance

• endurance

You may find these differ slightly depending on what you're reading but the overall aim remains the same – to increase muscle strength, prevent injury, give your heart a workout, and improve your core body stability, which is particularly relevant as you get older and are more prone to falls.

Gym phobic or gym bunny

Just getting through the doors of your local gym can seem like an endurance exercise. To the first-timer, fitness centres appear like another, scarier world, especially given the hi-tech machines with their red lights and rows of buttons to press. Plus the thought of working out in front of strangers who all look like they know what they're doing is even more stressful initially. You may be convinced everyone is staring at you like the new kid in the class at school.

Even now, I'm not entirely confident on exercise equipment, despite the best efforts of a personal trainer. But what I do know is that in reality your fellow gymgoers will be too focused on their own goals to notice what others around them are doing (or wearing). If anything, they'll appreciate the rookie, especially if you're carrying excess weight. That's because they know just how much harder you have to work to run on a treadmill when you're heavier.

Just to sound a note of caution here. At the point in my journey where I joined a gym, my weight was down to 15 stone (95kg), which was the result of adopting healthy eating habits and working out with my own trainer. It took preparation and planning to reach this stage, and I only did it when I knew I was ready. When I reached that point, I found a fitness centre as close to my flat in London as possible, so that I'd make use of it, and then buddy-ed up with their very experienced instructor who taught me the basics, such as how to use each piece of equipment safely and to maximum benefit. My first session with this fitness guru was daunting. However, there wasn't anything he pushed me to do that I wasn't capable of physically.

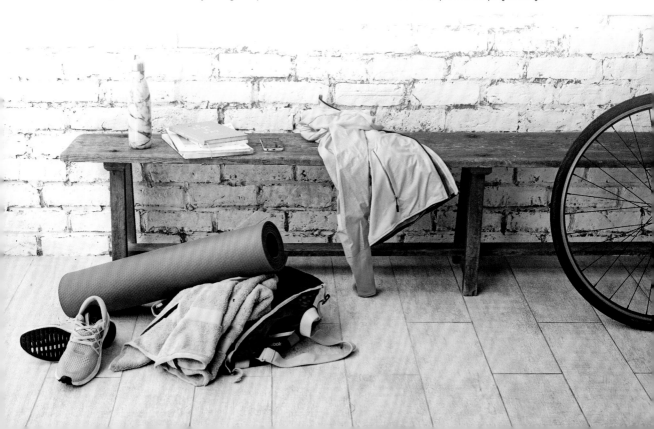

Zone 2

This may sound like the title for a sci-fi movie but Zone 2 exercise is the equivalent of a brisk walk. It means a level of fitness training that is just above easy. The main benefit of Zone 2 is that it builds on your aerobic capacity and with it your ability to maintain a faster pace for a longer period of time.

It's vigorous enough that if you tried to sing, you'd be out of breath, yet moderate enough to be able to just about hold a conversation. If this is as much exercise as you're able to do – and you can also wean yourself off sugar and processed food – then you'll be doing well. I did more than this but that doesn't mean you have to in order to switch from an unhealthy to a healthy lifestyle. It'll take longer, but you'll get there in the end. And if you carry on following this routine until you're well past retirement age, then you'll be laughing.

There are no hard and fast measurements with Zone 2 on what your maximum heart rate should be. If you're using a monitor, then it will probably be showing a target heart rate as 60–70% of your maximum heart rate – the fastest your heart is capable of beating safely. Exercising at maximum rate for every exercise session doesn't equal maximum efficiency. Instead, you could end up with sore joints. The secret is to find your 'sweet spot'. A fitness tracking device will calculate this for you, or you can work it out yourself with a simple calculation (see box below). A target heart rate should be in the region of 50–85% of maximum heart rate, and each type of workout should vary within this range according to how easy/strenuous it is.

How to work out your maximum heart rate and target exertion levels

- Write down your age, then subtract this figure from 220 to work out your maximum heart rate, for example 220 minus 50 years = 170 beats per minute

- Multiply the figure for your maximum heart rate by 50 then divide by 100 – this gives you a 50% exertion level, for example 50% of 170 = 85 beats per minute

- Multiply the figure for your maximum heart rate by 85 then divide by 100 – this gives you an 85% exertion level, for example 85% of 170 = 145 beats per minute

- So, the target heart rate for a 50-year-old to aim for during exercise is 85–145 beats per minute.

Resistance training

About a year into my downsizing odyssey, I felt as though my weight was plateauing. Don't get me wrong – by this point I was down to 15 stone (95kg), a weight I'd never imagined possible – but the truth was I had more fat to shift yet my progress had really slowed. The solution was to look to additional types of exercise to work into my now regular fitness routine. Which is where resistance training entered my life.

Resistance training or weight training is any exercise based around making your body work against a weight or a force by lifting/pulling with the aim of improving muscle strength. I turned to it to gain strength, muscle density and generally tighten bits of my body that needed it. There are also other, more unexpected, benefits of weight training. Building muscle mass enhances insulin sensitivity, as our bodies store carbs in two places – the liver and the muscles. For older people, this is particularly good news. A Japanese study found that when people in their sixties engaged in low-intensity resistance training they significantly improved their blood glucose levels.

Studies show, too, that regular weight training significantly reduces the risk of metabolic syndrome (see page 68). There are even studies that suggest lifting weights can head off dementia by stimulating production of brain cells. And if you're over 65, falls are a leading cause of death. Strengthening quads and glutes sees the risk of a fall drop by a third.

Perhaps best of all, there's just something about lifting weights that also lifts your mood. Numerous studies have shown that people who lift weights twice a week see significant reductions in the symptoms of depression. The theory is that lifting weights increases blood flow to the brain and releases mood-enhancing hormones such as norepinephrine and dopamine.

Resistance training is a type of exercise where a trainer can really help. They're particularly useful if you want to use weights but haven't done so before. My experience of resistance training was through signing up for a gym with a comprehensive selection of lifting equipment. It only took a few weeks for me to transition from being totally out of my comfort zone to lifting weights, doing squats and performing bench-presses. OK, so the results were hardly in the Arnold Schwarzenegger league (or even Popeye for that matter), but I felt so much fitter and stronger.

Personal trainers

So many people join gyms in January for a New Year resolution then never go back. Or in June when they're thinking of how they'll look on the beach. If you join a gym, make sure you fix up with one of their instructors who can help work out a programme for you and set aside time in your week to actually use the facilities. Otherwise, you may as well burn your hard-earned money.

Another option is hiring your own personal trainer, as I did, for weekly sessions, but this depends on how much you have to spend. If you've not got the budget, then don't worry – you can achieve your downsizing goals without a trainer.

However, if you have the income available, personal trainers are a great value-for-money proposition, as I found with mine. Their job is to help you leave the building fitter and stronger and they'll get you to that point faster by teaching you techniques, giving you confidence, and knowing when you're having a good/bad day. They're an asset if you want to increase your gains from exercise.

That first morning, when I staggered out of bed at 5.30am for my debut session with my trainer Clayton will be forever etched in my memory. My kit had been selected from the bargain bin of the local sports shop, my trainers were more than a decade old and I was a bag of nerves. But despite all this, it felt like a chance to start again and to leave behind the old Tom.

At points during this first workout, I confess to feeling light-headed, weak, humiliated and very vulnerable. The thought of quitting was never far from my mind. But by the time I got home, the feeling of elation was intense after the 22-stone (140kg) me had achieved:

• Warm-up exercises, including knee bends and side stretches

• Press ups (two in total) and only using a park bench

• Jumps on and off an 8-inch-high ledge of a children's sandpit (15 in total)

• Runs backwards and forwards across a 3-foot-high miniature bridge

Over time, these workouts became less of an ordeal. To my surprise, I even began to find I was enjoying them, although Clayton ensured he kept increasing the challenge to keep me on my toes. We began incorporating other routines into the sessions, such as boxercise, where I'd pummel vinyl pads as hard as possible while bouncing on my feet constantly.

Remember, this was all played out in a public space so there was an embarrassment factor initially which disappeared once I became more confident.

For me, the benefits of hiring a trainer were many and included:

- **Focus** – having a regular slot in your diary boosts your motivation and makes it harder to shirk your exercise commitments.

- **Bespoke approach** – a trainer has the knowledge to devise a varied regime based on your abilities, such as the boxercise. This takes the stress out of having to figure it out yourself.

- **Personal development** – they assess your movement and agility, then improve on these, pushing you further and nudging you when you fall behind.

How to find a personal trainer

Like any relationship, it has to work or you won't feel the benefits, won't put the effort in and will end up feeling miserable. You should always be prepared to move on and find someone new, if necessary. The best method for finding a trainer is word of mouth – that's how I found Clayton. Or you could check out the National Register of Personal Trainers: www.nrpt.co.uk.

- **Sleep and nutrition** – these are key elements of a healthy lifestyle. Your personal trainer will analyse these and advise you on sensible changes to make.

- **Reassurance** – a trainer provides psychological as well as physical support. For me, it was almost like having a therapist because there's nothing they've not heard before when it comes to weight and fitness woes.

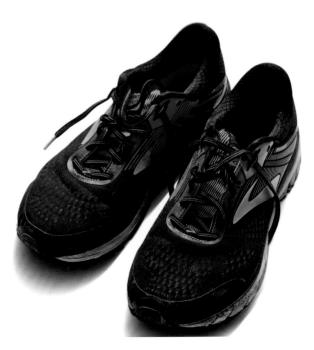

High-intensity interval training (HIIT)

I spent the last chapter explaining that you don't need to turn yourself into a trembling mass of sweating and hyperventilating exhaustion to change your life. If you downsize correctly, though, your desire to change yourself will be so great that you will have foregone your old lifestyle and will be looking for new and rewarding challenges. I love HIIT. I hate HIIT. Welcome to HIIT! Sometimes I can consistently train at this level, other times my mental fortitude fails me. My fitness journey will forever be a work in progress.

So what exactly is High-Intensity Interval Training? Essentially, it is a method of stretching your body to the limit for a very brief period of time, usually within a 15-minute session.

HIIT boosts aerobic and cardiac activity with the aim of improving your resilience – your body becomes able to perform more energetic exercise for longer by being stressed to discomfort and then recovering. The way I worked it into my exercise regime was by going on a very light jog, then sprinting as fast as I could for 20 seconds three times during my run. Going as fast as I could left me gulping for air but it was only for 20 seconds, then my pounding heart would return to its normal rate.

The NHS Couch to 5K programme features elements of interval training. The plan was developed by a self-confessed running hater, Josh Clark, who wanted to help his mum get off the couch and change his own perception of running as torture. A running plan for total novices, Couch to 5K combines walking with brief bursts of running, eventually building up to longer running sessions to meet the 5km target. The app is free and easy to download and features coaching from celebrities including Jo Whiley and Sarah Millican, or you can tune into the Couch to 5K podcasts.

Or you could try CAROL, which delivers a high-intensity workout in the living room and is regarded as the ultimate in 'smart' stationary exercise bikes. The equivalent of a Ferrari or Aston Martin for fitness nerds, CAROL stands for 'cardiovascular optimisation logic' and is equipped with an artificial intelligence (AI) system that tailors each ride to the individual.

The concept is based on the theory that short bursts or doses of high-intensity exercise – starting with two 20-second sprints in the case of CAROL – rapidly depletes your muscles of glycogen (a form of glucose stored by the body). If forced to adjust, your body becomes more efficient at turning to fat as an energy source once glycogen runs low. This relates back to what I explained in the earlier section on diets (see page 50) and how low-carb diets are aimed at getting your body to turn to burning fat once you've exhausted your glycogen stores.

The makers of this at-home bike claim that it delivers the benefits of a 45-minute run in less than a minute. Each time you use the bike, the computer system analyses your data to calculate the exact resistance you need to be pushed to reach new targets. The sessions gradually become more demanding. You will be feeling the pressure once you have done around half a dozen workouts and your fitness is improving.

Of course, you could argue that the downside is not getting the added benefits of being outside in the fresh air and green spaces. You also need to be feeling flush as CAROL will set you back more than £2,000.

Injuries

If you're over 50, then working out and exercising can take its toll on your joints and bones. Ageing leads to the bones becoming thinner and weaker, a process triggered by the body reabsorbing existing bone cells faster than it can make new bone.

And muscle mass reduces, too, as a result of several factors, such as a decline in the body's messengers (motor neurons) which control muscles. The less muscle, the less protection for bones. Lifting too much and with a poor technique is a recipe for injury whatever your age.

So often you see people in gyms who clearly haven't been taught the correct technique for handling weights, etc. Doing movements your body isn't used to or which exert force on the wrong muscles can end in disaster.

Cycling isn't without its hazards either, whether that's in the form of shouty lorry drivers, impatient car drivers or saddle sores. If you do a safety course (see page 114, for more details on these), then hopefully these won't be in the form of a road accident.

Scrapes and bruises are inevitable though, as I found out on my first long-distance rural outing when I had an unfortunate encounter with a tractor and ended up with a gash in my leg and in lying a nettle-filled ditch.

The message I'm giving you here is always warm up your body before exercising, keep hydrated, wear the right kit and ask the advice of an expert if attempting strenuous activity.

Top common fitness injuries

- Shoulder pain
- Knee pain related to physical activity (for example, knee ligament sprains)
- Hip and groin pain
- Muscle injuries
- Activity-related tendon problems (for example, knees, wrists)
- Ankle ligament sprains
- Ankle pain
- Exertional lower leg pain (shin splints)
- Sport-related back pain

Cycling

Once I'd worked out my exercise regime, it finally dawned on me that I didn't need a car when I lived in a city – I could cycle instead and keep fit at the same time. Let's face it, no one gets fit sat in traffic holding on to a steering wheel. So, the car went, which also saved me a fortune in tax and insurance and more than covered the cost of gym membership and my growing collection of gym gear.

Next, I went to retrieve the Trek hybrid bike I'd bought in an impulsive moment, only to abandon it in the shed in the back garden of the house I rented a room in just off the Old Kent Road in London. The cycle had become a home for every spider in the neighbourhood. The first hurdle to overcome was losing enough weight to fit on a bike in the first place. The second was overcoming my anxiety about cycling around a traffic-choked London with confidence, instead of fearing I'd be knocked off every time I ventured out.

Learning safe cycling

In the UK, headlines about cyclists who have been knocked off their bikes are a tragic and all-too-common reality these days. Some councils should be praised for improving access for cyclists with dedicated lanes to make their journeys safer. Others are ignoring the issue. That's why learning how to keep safe is essential through courses like Bikeability, which is the modern version of what was the Cycling Proficiency Test. Not riding too close to the kerb, surveying your road space properly and being decisive turning left/right at junctions were among the many invaluable tips I learned while on this course. Find more information at www.bikeability.org.uk.

One of the best and most useful things I did was to sign up to a Bikeability safe cycling course (see box above). It only took a few hours of lessons and by the end of them I was able to navigate the roundabout in Trafalgar Square without ending up white-knuckled and sweaty-palmed.

I want to ride a bicycle – but which one?

Take time to do your research and speak to staff in specialist cycling shops. When it came to choosing my bike, the Trek was very reliable for my initial forays onto the streets of London and I became very fond of its ability to get me from A to B without too much trouble. Not only was it an excellent mode of transport, the Trek also became the focus for my system of goals and rewards to help me lose more weight, as I outlined earlier (see page 36). Over time, however, it became apparent that it was the equivalent of a first romance and we were starting to outgrow one another. Now I'd gained my cycling 'spurs', I was eager to take part

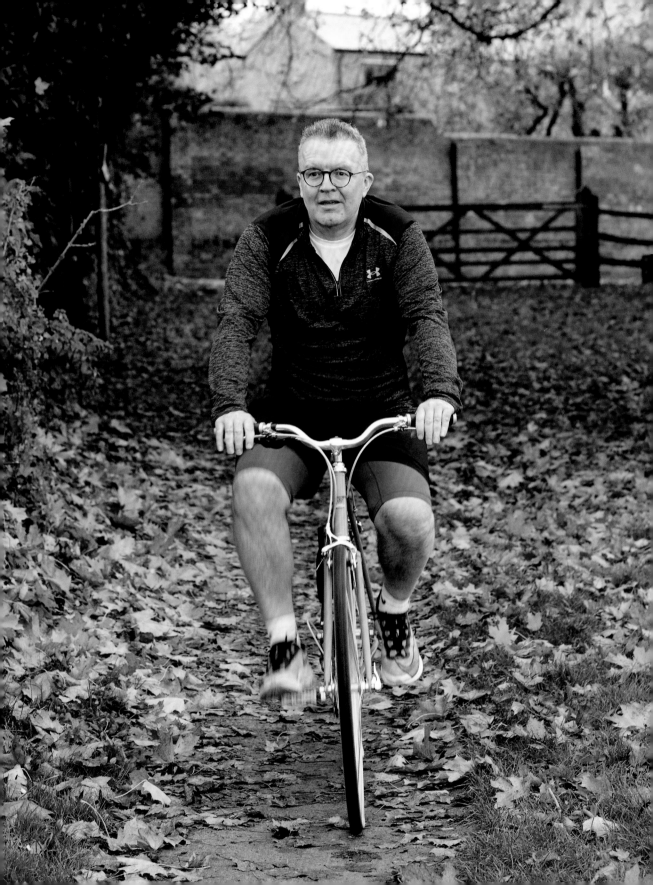

Cycling essentials

- Helmet that is a proper fit

- Padded shorts (your bottom/crotch will thank you!)

- Lights

- Gloves

- Water bottle

- Flat tyre repair kit

In the world of e-biking, a VanMoof is up there with the best if you're into technology. The rider has an app to control the speed of the bike as well as an alarm and security tracker to prevent your two-wheeled vehicle getting stolen. If you're new to biking, though, my choices would be:

Good starter
Trek Hybrid

Better road bike
Focus Izalco

Best for everyday commuting
VanMoof e-bike

in some team challenges, for which I'd need a nippier set of wheels. What's more, I'd set myself a symbolic milestone of losing 100lb (45.4kg) in weight in return for treating myself to a brand-new model, a sleek Focus Izalco.

My next and current 'relationship' is with an e-bike, which is essentially like an ordinary bike but with an electric motor added that's powered by a battery. There's been a real revolution in e-bikes, which means they now offer something for everyone. The price may seem off-putting but you will end up saving money over time, especially if you live in the suburbs and commute to work. I chose a VanMoof bike as it's a company that focuses solely on City commuter biking. Another bonus is you don't end up dripping with sweat after riding one because the motor means you have to make less effort pedalling, particularly up hills. OK, you may not burn as many calories as you would on a conventional bike but you're still getting a decent workout and increasing your heart rate. They're certainly not the lazy person's option (or cheating) – they won't work unless you do the work first. You can pedal them like a regular bike, then use the electric assistance when things get really tough and you're in a hurry.

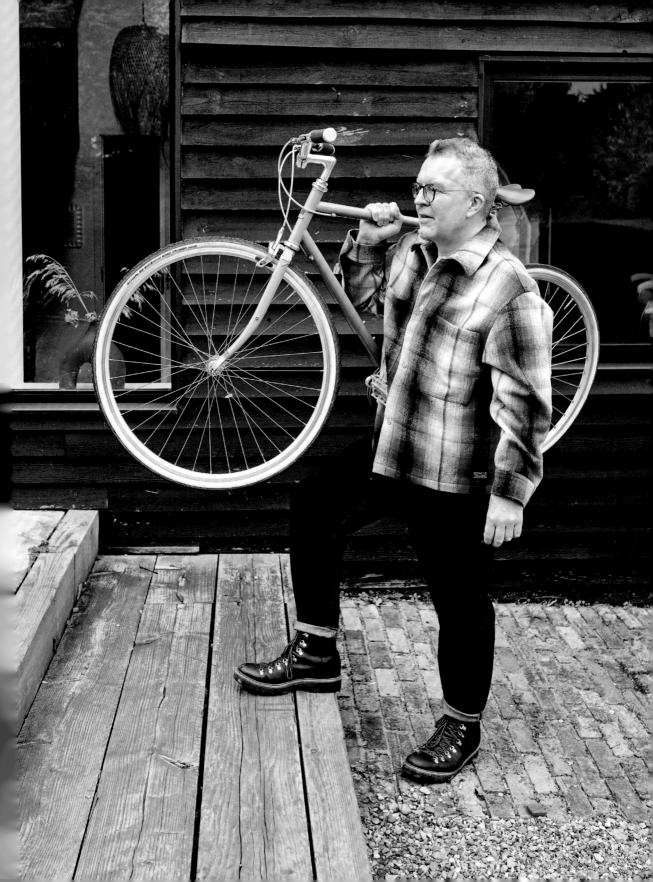

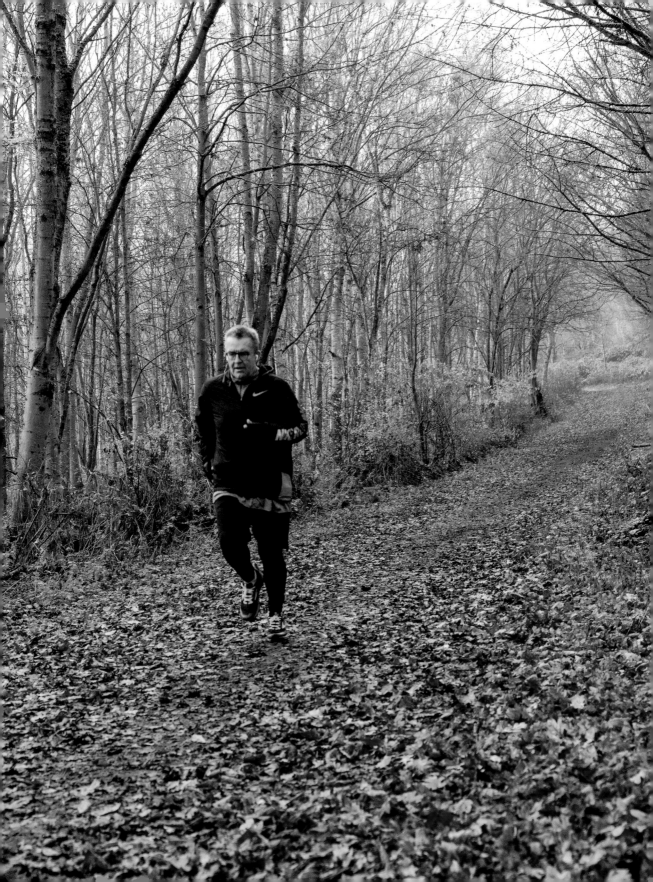

Several studies have shown that e-bikes are capable of providing much of the cardiovascular benefits associated with conventional bicycles. Research published in the journal *JMIR Public Health and Surveillance,* based on 33 adults aged 19–28, found that the mean average heart rate was only 6.21 beats lower over a 10-mile ride compared with cycling the same distance on a conventional bike. However, both sets of results were significantly higher than resting heart rate. Another study by US researchers published only recently came to a similar conclusion and found that the intensity level provided by an e-bike met those recommended by the World Health Organization for physical activity.

IN SUMMARY

- The less you move, the more sedentary you are, the less the body removes fat from your body, which can lead to clogged arteries and strokes, so incorporate movement into your daily routine, conducting meetings as you walk, for example.

- Daily steps will help you hit the World Health Organization target of 150 minutes a week of moderate-intensity physical activity, that is, exercise that boosts your heart rate, such as climbing stairs or gardening.

- Aim for 5,000 steps at day at the start of your journey (the equivalent of 4km or 2.5 miles), and accept that walking more is a lifelong mission to maintain your weight (not a short-term fix). Raise your steps target when 5,000 steps becomes easy.

- Hitting the gym on day one of your downsizing programme will end in failure – get your cupboards, schedules and routines in place first.

- If you take up cycling, research the type of bike to buy and think about investing in an e-bike to get you around faster while still burning calories – and do a cycle safety course so you're fit for the road.

- Don't overdo it – the golden rule if you're over 50 is to avoid injuries.

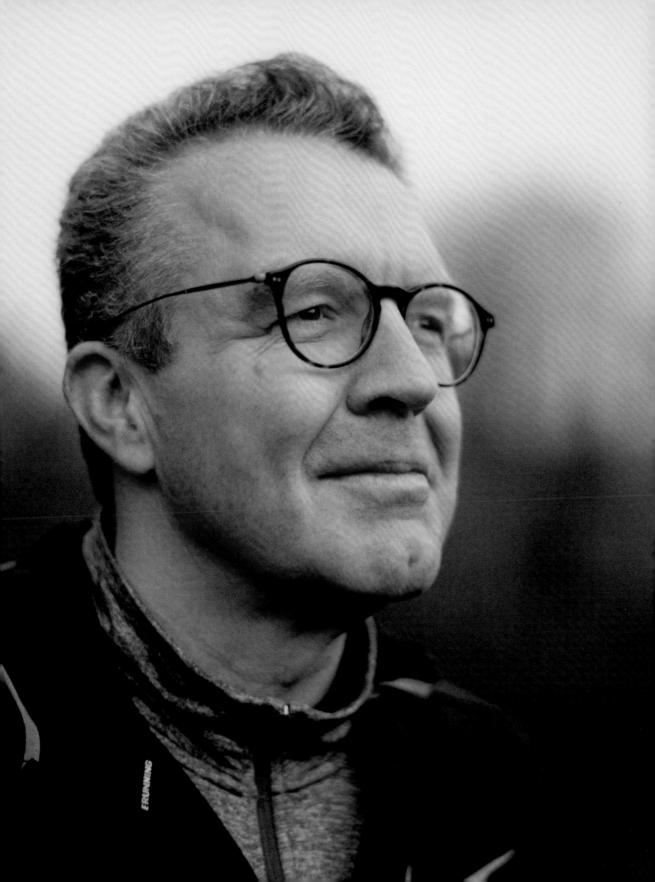

5 Maintenance

We're all human. One day you're going to wake up, your trousers will feel a bit tight, and you'll be horrified to find you've put on half a stone (3kg) without noticing the weight has been creeping back on. You'll realise you've been out more and drunk more, and so the guilt sets in. Most likely, it won't be one incident – there will be many tiny slips that have gradually led to this. Either that or a major lifestyle change. When you reach this moment, the first key message is not to panic. And don't punish yourself or go into denial. The greatest challenge of downsizing is keeping the excess pounds off long term, with some studies showing that more than half of weight loss is regained within two years. When you find yourself in this situation, what's needed is a reset programme to reapply some of the basic rules of downsizing, reinforce positive behaviour and address negative habits.

For me, three and a half years of progress was almost sabotaged by three and a half months of falling off the weight-loss wagon. I'd come so far and shed so much only to put a stone and a half back on. What was hard to deal with was the fact I was now conscious of the harm I was doing to my health. The 'old' (obese) me had been blissfully ignorant until my diabetes diagnosis.

Thankfully, I had not completely lost my control. My inner voice kept asking how this setback in my journey could possibly have happened in the first place? How could I have reached the top of the mountain both figuratively and then literally, and then lost my footing? The truth is that I had drifted and taken a wrong turn, in part because of the monumental curveball that has been the COVID-19 pandemic, which coincided with some major shifts in my personal circumstances.

There I was living in London, doing the same job, and following a routine that got me results – my daily steps, my runs and my gym sessions. The next minute my work and life pattern changed completely. I moved to a different part of the country and was no longer a Member of Parliament. Before I knew it, my entire regime just collapsed and disorder took its place. Like millions of other people, I found myself in lockdown and spending all my waking hours sat in a chair in my home office. All those opportunities I'd enjoyed (or at the time cursed) to incorporate activity into my daily life had disappeared overnight.

To add to all this, the place where I was now living was bang in the middle of the countryside. One of the biggest myths is that being surrounded by green space equals being fitter. Dog owners may benefit because they have to take their pet out at least twice a day, whatever the weather, or risk ending up with a seriously miserable and hyperactive pooch. But the reality of rural living is that you need transport to get around, and two wheels are only suitable for trips that don't include picking up friends from the station, visiting DIY stores or travelling to do a family shop.

Another issue is the lack of places to park your bike. There are more than 20,000 spaces alone at stations across London, but it's a different story when you live outside a big city. A lot of towns haven't caught up with cities in providing the infrastructure which would make cycling easier. There was no longer a Tube to hop on to (and escalators to walk up and down). Instead, it meant me having to buy a second-hand car in order to be able to travel around or visit people – and no one gets fit driving a car. Don't get me wrong, I'm not ungrateful for living in a beautiful part of England surrounded by fields and green spaces, especially during COVID-19 when city-dwellers were cooped up in flats with no gardens or had to share overcrowded parks.

Another consequence I'd not considered as a result of changing my lifestyle was the mental impact of losing a routine that had taken months to establish. In lockdown three, my daily average steps fell to around 2,500 a day vs the 10,000 I'd been so proud to achieve. My morale was starting to plummet, and I was waking up anxious, fearing that I would end up back as that person I'd tried so hard to escape. The question that played constantly on my mind was 'Is this the unwelcome return of Tommy Two Dinners?'

It took me a while to adapt and work out how I could incorporate cycling and exercise into my daily routine. I had to go back and dust off my downsizing blueprint. Looking at your priorities is useful too when you reset. Do you have a good work/life balance? What really matters to you? Are your family happy and healthy, and are you truly present in their lives? These are among the questions I'd suggest you ask yourself.

Routine reset

Life is a series of episodes. Sooner or later, you will be on to the next phase with all the new experiences and challenges this brings. It could be a big shift that throws you off balance, such as moving house and changing job (as I did) or a more subtle one, such as realising that an older relative needs you to be around more to support them. Career changes, family health issues – any of these issues can disrupt the daily routine that normally you would rely on to set you up for the day.

In chapter one, I highlighted how habits are made up of tiny behaviours and rules. Actions such as using your lunch break to fit in a walk may sound obvious or trivial but we often don't realise how they add up to a whole way of living. Routines are an essential part of your downsizing programme and also of a health reset. When you physically move to a different environment or are faced with a new mental hurdle, then many of the things you take for granted – your exercise spot or buddy who runs with you – can disappear, often overnight.

This can play havoc with your ability to maintain a healthy weight, despite all your best efforts. Everyone has setbacks, so what you need is a reset. To try to rebuild your

Week one reset

- Food logging and daily weighing should be top of your priority list, along with measuring your step count. (You can add in blood sugar level and ketone measurements if it helps.)

- Prepare yourself mentally – don't let your mood spiral because your activity levels are non-existent, your weight is up and so is your carb count.

- Focus just on each day in week one, then at the end reflect on what might have led to weight gain in the previous months. Have you created an unconscious bad habit perhaps? Mine was ordering cheese during lockdown. Six weeks later and I realised I was eating four times as much blooming cheese than I had prior to lockdown.

habits, set little rules again that are easy to keep and that when taken as a whole have a big impact over time. Remember that can of fizzy drink I talked about? Choosing not to drink it once is great, but choosing not to drink it every day for a year brings amazing results. The same applies with your daily steps: going back to reset and doing 2,000 more steps a day adds up to 730,000 over a year.

The positive news was that this time round I was also more aware of my bad habits and what needed to change. Everything I had learned about myself, and my own behaviour, had not been wasted because I'd taken the time to lay down routines that worked. What this meant was that I was equipped with the tools and the right mindset to pick myself up and start again, however dispiriting this was at first. So ingrained was my knowledge and training that I had these resources into which I could dig down deep.

Be honest with yourself

Consider the following scenario. You always put your trainers in the shoe rack by the front door so when you go for a walk you know where to find them. But you've moved house and they're in a different place entirely and you keep forgetting where that place is. Or they're somewhere in a box that you keep meaning to go and open.

Or does the following sound familiar? You've changed jobs so you're now too far from the gym you used to visit in the morning before work. You tell yourself you'll find a new place but somehow you just never get the time to check out the options.

There are a million books out there on lifestyle changes. About the shirt colour you should wear or how to fold your socks. What you actually need is a system check to analyse how to organise your days and weeks and establish if your habits and routines are productive in achieving your goals. This has to be consciously thought about.

A routine that's malfunctioning or collapsed is the equivalent of a system failure, a problem or slip up to be solved instead of a disaster. It counts as a setback, as does a week in meltdown because you've not exercised enough. Failure, on the other hand, is when you've reached the point where you've chosen not to carry on because you've put on too much weight and resetting the psychological dial is too overwhelming.

Don't let a setback turn into failure, a point of no return. Every day there are issues we face and following a downsizing programme is no different – you could get a flat bike tyre, the piece of equipment you want to use at the gym could be occupied or you've gone out for a walk without a coat and it starts pouring. The issue is how do you deal with you. For 35 years, I dealt with it by ignoring the sensible voice in my head or compounding my system failings by defying logic. Downsizing isn't a finite thing. Be clear with yourself that this is a journey without end and there are ups and downs. When you have a little slip, use it to reset.

I'd been doing a Zoom meeting at a particular time every week. When I did my reset, I realised it was a barrier to getting in my steps. The solution? I asked the team if we could do the call when I was out on my daily walk instead, and they agreed. You could call that courtesy in a digital age, but it's an example of identifying what's now stopping you from achieving your goals and finding a way forward. With other calls, my strategy has been to ditch the office chair I hardly left during lockdown (except to eat or sleep) and replace it with an exercise ball to give my core muscles (including my pelvic, abdominal and lower back muscles) a workout. Or I move around the house when I'm on the phone to get in some more of those precious daily steps. The downside is your family may get a little irritated but the benefit your body gets is worth the price of the odd glare now and again.

Often, when you take a moment to analyse what they are, the reasons behind barriers can be very simple. Like when I joined a gym and didn't realise towels were not provided, which meant spending the rest of the day soaked in my sweat. It sounds trivial but it was a setback that could have easily turned into failure if I'd let it. Now I always check out what I need to bring and make sure I'm prepared before setting off.

My personal reset plan

- Signing up to my nearest fitness centre once gyms reopened last April (2021). For me, this was not only about fitness but about controlling my food input because they provide work areas (away from my home fridge).

- Writing a reset plan that maps out daily nutrition, activity and exercise. This is about managing my productive time and measuring progress for which MyFitnessPal app is vital. Going back to my gratitude journaling to bank new wins.

- Booking a personal trainer twice a week for focus and accountability and to brush up on my exercise technique.

- Getting my bike serviced and putting it in a place where I can easily access it.

- Dusting off and recharging the weighing scales.

- Locking behavioural change back into my routine. This was to limit the mental barriers to being active once again, such as finding a separate box for my gym kit and putting my running socks at the top of the clothes drawer.

Before you slide too far, have an honest conversation with yourself. Try asking yourself these questions:

- Why am I not following my usual movement/eating/sleep regime?

- What do I need to give up to make time to exercise?

- How can I organise my diary better to make room for cooking a healthy dinner?

- What can I do to make sure I remember my towel for the gym/my water bottle/my activity tracker?

One of my routes back to reset was to identify a new walking route in the area where I now live. It was the first step to getting myself out of the house again and re-establishing my routine. The next was to sort through my kit to see what did/didn't fit, and what needed replacing. Thinking about where best to put the scales was important. They had been in the bathroom in the new house but that wasn't working and this created a mental barrier to me using them. It was a case of 'out of sight, out of mind'. Now they sit under a cupboard in the kitchen near the place I make the coffee so I can't ignore them.

Getting positive support

Your weight-loss journey may be lonely at the start. But you won't be alone for long. What you'll discover is that others will be willing you on and will be amazingly generous. It could be those in the exercise class you take up or other members of the running club you join. Or even your adversaries. Some of my harshest political opponents would discuss running techniques with me and how hard it was eating proper food, and even made positive comments about my slimmed-down frame. Whether it's from your new weight-loss networks or your existing friendship circle, you'll discover who these cheerleaders are (and also who to avoid). Hold on to them and turn to them when the journey gets tough. My first proper slump was winter 2020. Turning to the gym wasn't an option – it was lockdown so they were closed. Instead, the first thing I did was to contact my accountability group. I've now set up an official app which you can find under my name in the App Store. The Persons of Positivity (POP) club provides live broadcasts, fitness challenges or just a place to hang out and chat about healthy lifestyles.

The support club developed out of posts I made on Facebook and conversations with my followers about my need to get back on track. It turned out that most of them were in the same situation and needed to set new targets. What came from this was an app, a community of people including friends who support each other in their goal to improve their weight. If you want to join, then you can download my app on the App Store (search for 'Tom Watson').

Before the pandemic hit in 2020, I was running 5km every day with this group only then for my activity levels to barely hit 5km in an average week during the dark February days of 2021. Being upfront with friends, family and my POP group – sharing the lows as well as the highs – is a fundamental part of being honest with myself in order to continue on the lifelong journey of maintaining a healthy and active lifestyle. After all, it was my self-deception about the harm I was doing to myself that resulted in my type 2 diabetes diagnosis. The advice POP members sent me included:

- Set a mini target of 3km walking a day.

- Clear your diary again for exercise.

- Phone your accountability partner on your daily walk.

Quit the snacking

Earlier on in this book, I talked about the importance of food logging when you first start out on your weight-loss journey. I was quite obsessive about monitoring my nutrient

Let me share a couple of 'Tom tips' here:

- Never eat directly from the fridge. Take a moment to ask yourself if you need a plate for the food you're taking out. Or better still, always put whatever you're taking out on to a plate, even if it's a few carrot sticks dipped into a keto mayonnaise. Otherwise, several trips later and you'll find that you have eaten the equivalent of a meal. And never eat anything with your hands – always make yourself get a knife and fork. As with using a plate, this technique may make you think twice about raiding the fridge.

- Don't con yourself about how much you're snacking when you're around someone else's house or at a social function. Even one crisp is a chink in your 'armour' – this form of eating is part of the denial process and leads to unhealthy habits forming.

intake but became more relaxed as the pounds fell off and my discipline grew. If bad habits do creep in, then returning to food logging is a good idea. A home office 12 feet from the kitchen led to my weight gain in lockdown. Aside from the cheese obsession, late-night snacking was largely to blame for bad habits developing – those visits to the fridge after 8pm 'Just to see what's there'. It's almost like a reflex action for me: I don't really know I'm doing it, especially when I'm talking on the phone at the same time. But it's my weak point, which I will always have to monitor.

Many major paid-for weight-loss programmes include maintenance as part of their package. WeightWatchers, for example, will monitor your weight every week to ensure you're keeping on track. It can be reassuring to feel that you've got that support. The flaw in this is that once you leave the programme it's too easy to fall into your bad old ways and pile on the weight.

By all means buddy up with others if that helps you to stay disciplined. But always remember you're the one responsible for keeping count of your own pounds/kilos, and this has to be done on a daily basis when you hit the reset button.

Through devising my own reboot, I gradually got back into a new routine and back to the 'Tom' who does 10,000 steps a day. Not the 'Tom' who eats food off other people's plates. What I've not mentioned here is the importance of self-nurture, which includes sleep and mental wellbeing.

Self-nurture

A dial reset is more likely to succeed if you make yourself a priority and truly believe your body and wellbeing is worth looking after. Many people will be reading this and thinking how is this possible when they're overloaded with responsibilities, an endless to-do list and what seems like not enough hours in the day to achieve all this. Sleep and self-care are all too often the casualties of the constant battle to fit in work, domestic chores, time with family and maintaining a social life.

I hear you. Life is a daily struggle of juggling commitments and this Covid-era has added an extra layer of complexity that we're all still navigating our way around. Lockdowns, social distancing, not being able to hug friends – these are all challenges imposed by these exceptional times and they have left millions feeling isolated, anxious and unable to look forward or plan. Others, including NHS and care staff, have worked on the frontline throughout and are close to – or already experiencing – burnout.

We're not robots, despite our increasing interaction with and reliance on technology. We're human beings (not human 'doings'). In the chapter on mindset, I touched on techniques to promote a more positive mental attitude. These will not only help you in your downsizing goals but also make you more resilient to what life throws at you.

Make sure you take time to analyse and understand how stress affects your relationship with food. Did I consume more when I was under pressure or feeling unable to cope? Absolutely, sometimes in the form of a jumbo bar of milk chocolate. Resorting to over-eating as a form of comfort is a common response to stressful situations. This form of self-soothing or self-medicating is based on the way sugar stimulates the brain's reward system, possibly even more so than class A drugs such as cocaine.

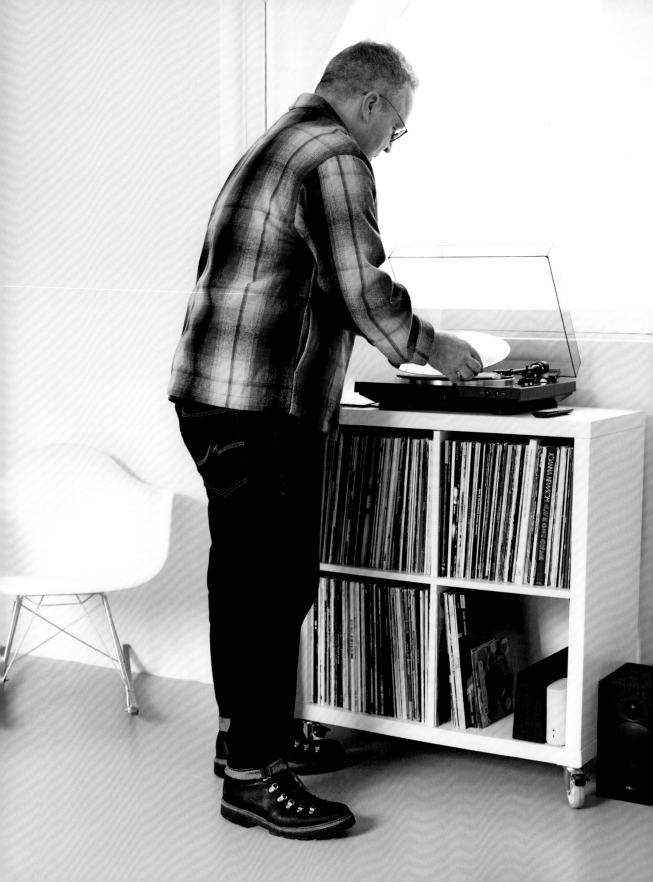

Setting a sleep pattern

What is also key is a healthy sleep pattern. Having monitored my weight obsessively during my downsizing journey, I know the weight never drops off when I've had a restless night. In my experience, sleep is top of the list as far as essential ingredients for good health are concerned, followed by nutrition, exercise and wellbeing. So give yourself the *right* to 8 hours' sleep. That's the optimum amount, say many scientists, including Professor Matthew Walker, director of the Center for Human Sleep Science at the University of California, and author of *Why We Sleep*. To me, good-quality sleep is the equivalent of medicine or, in the words of Professor Walker, 'emotional first aid'.

According to Professor Walker, we're in the middle of a sleep-loss epidemic and our lack of shut-eye is linked to obesity, diabetes, cancer and Alzheimer's. Increased light pollution, technology on constantly in the bedroom and the erosion of boundaries between work and free time have all contributed to this crisis, he says. You've all probably heard the claim that Margaret Thatcher survived on just 4 hours' sleep on weekdays. Or even Napoleon's habit of sleeping between midnight and 2am, then again between 5am and 7am. Well, scientists have now identified genes associated with natural short sleep patterns that last 4–6 hours but leaves those with it feeling well-rested. This is the exception, not the rule – the vast majority of us end up cranky and exhausted if we have to survive on so few hours. Professor Walker also blames a macho culture surrounding sleep where anyone needing the full 8 hours is perceived to be weak, despite the fact that in reality no one can survive on 5 hours or less without suffering the consequences. This attitude is sadly prevalent among some at Westminster, although growing awareness around mental health means it is starting to change.

Before my downsizing journey, late nights were a regular – sometimes daily feature – of my life as an MP and I never had a standard bedtime. There was all the paperwork that comes with the job of being an MP, and which I'd be going through until the small hours, the need to attend late-night votes in the Commons, and the email briefings that would arrive before dawn and had to be responded to before breakfast. Life on the campaign trail meant a maximum of 6 hours snatched head-on-pillow time thanks to overheated hotel rooms. To add to my sleep deprivation, I'd also stay up playing video games. Or socialising – Luigi Polledri was like family to me given all the time I spent in his Soho restaurant, Little Italy.

My poor night-time habits didn't bode well for my long-term physical health, including my weight. I'm pretty sure that my disrupted circadian rhythm was a significant factor in my insulin resistance, my high blood pressure and my obesity. Even when I did get to bed, I'd wake up through the night to go to the toilet, an early warning sign (although I didn't know it then) of diabetes. And then there was my snoring, another symptom of being overweight. Waking up feeling jaded was such a frequent occurrence that I thought nothing of it, let

> Sleep regenerates the brain, boosts the immune system and reduces the risk of infection.

alone linked it to the fact that I was officially sleep deprived, which is defined as getting less than 7 hours at a time.

Professor Luigi Fontana (see page 70) says sleep regenerates the brain, improves the efficiency of the immune system and reduces the risk of infections, while also playing a vital role in consolidating memories and reducing the risk of dementia. As long as you get good-quality sleep, there is no magic number of hours for everyone, in his opinion. The most important thing is that sleep is deep and restful and you wake feeling restored. That's where strategies to improve sleep quality, such as endurance exercise, yoga and meditation, can be useful.

The first step I took to tackle my toxic sleeping habits was to set myself a regular bedtime of between 9 and 10pm. Before making this small but hugely significant change, I'd wake up feeling achy, in pain and not knowing where I was. This new routine combined with regular exercise (which tired me out naturally) resulted in me starting the day feeling refreshed and more able to face what was in store. I used to crawl out of bed. These days I leap.

Why regular sleep is vital for good health

Circadian rhythms regulate our 24-hour sleep-wake cycle and are influenced by cues such as light. Epidemiological studies have reported that shift work in particular is related to a risk of diseases such as cancer because of the effect on circadian rhythms. If the rhythms are disrupted, your sleep is too, and this impacts on physical and mental health. After just one bad night, natural killer cells – those that keep diseases at bay such as cancer – drop dramatically. Adults aged 45 years or older who sleep less than 6 hours a night have a much greater risk of dying from a heart attack or stroke in their lifetime. This is compared with those getting 7 or 8 hours a night. Blood pressure is partly to blame – just one night of modest sleep reduction will speed up a person's heart rate and raise blood pressure. A lack of sleep also appears to sabotage effective blood sugar control. In experiments, the cells of the sleep-deprived have been shown to become less responsive to insulin. When your sleep becomes short, this makes the body more susceptible to weight gain. Reasons include a drop in the hormone leptin, which inhibits hunger, and a rise in levels of ghrelin, which is associated with appetite.

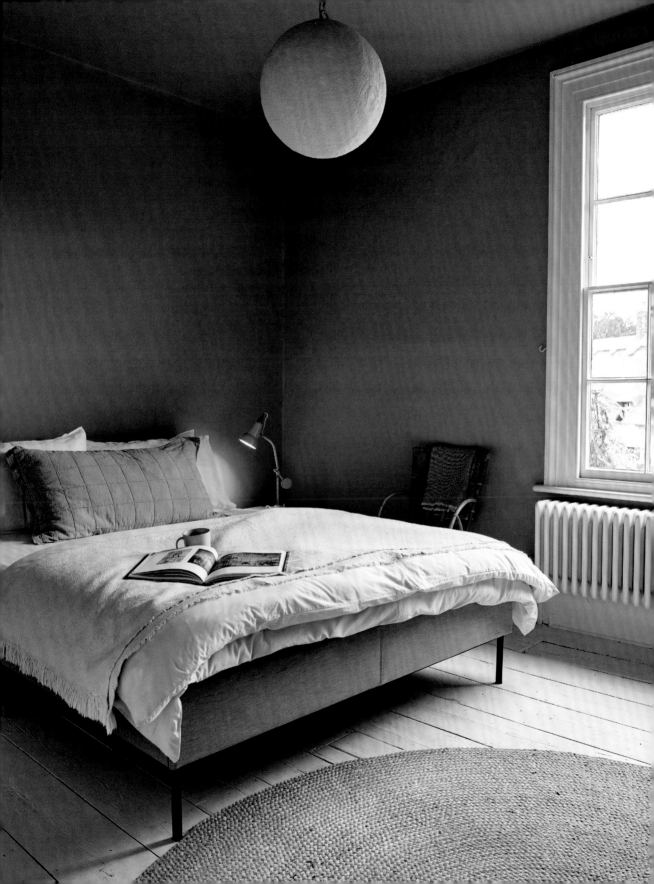

Improving your sleep habits
Good
Write down the time you go to bed/when you get up

Better
Get a sleep app

Best
Invest in a wearable device that measures sleep, such as an Oura Ring

Studies suggest the light from digital screens blocks the sleep-inducing hormone melatonin.

Going sugar-free also had a knock-on effect on my sleep because I was no longer waking up i|n the night to go and pee once my blood sugar levels had come down. The snoring also improved once the weight began to come off, which not only benefited me from a sleep viewpoint but I'm sure my neighbours breathed a sigh of relief too.

Not drinking or eating just before bed makes a major difference. I measure my sleep using a special gadget called an Oura Ring. This looks like a wedding band but can be made to fit on any finger, and it tells me useful information such as how many hours I'm getting, how deep the sleep is, as well as my body temperature and heart rate through the night. What I've noticed is that my resting heart rate increases by about 10 beats a minute above my average if I've had just one glass of wine, and it's even higher when I eat heavily. Eating later than 6pm would lead to more erratic and disturbed sleep than normal, particularly during the rapid eye movement (REM) phase when the learning, memory and mood regions of the brain are being stimulated. All this data and more was a complete revelation to me, and the sleep ring has become an indispensable part of my wellbeing plan.

Apart from the sleep 'disruptors' that we consume, there are many physical barriers that can be eliminated or minimised. Your laptop, TV and other digital screens all emit blue LED light, which messes with your rest because some studies suggest it blocks the sleep-inducing hormone melatonin. And light receptors in the eyes are most sensitive to this blue light, which has very short but high-energy wavelengths. Exposure during the day to blue light (the largest source is sunlight) helps maintain a healthy circadian rhythm by keeping us alert. At night, it disturbs our wake-and-sleep cycle. Device manufacturers have attempted to reduce blue light emissions at night from devices such as iPads, but a study by experts in the US found that the interventions they've come up with aren't enough to prevent the suppression of melatonin. If you can, turn off your iPhone and other gadgets in the bedroom so you can't be disturbed by blue LED light. If that's not possible, make sure you don't access social media or go roaming around on Google – and *don't* scroll through emails in the middle of the night (remember what I said about a right to sleep).

Here are some other tips I found useful when setting a slumber regime:

- Declutter your bedroom – it should be a sanctuary, not an overflow office.

- Switch to blackout blinds on your windows – or line your curtains with them.

- Get new pillows to improve your comfort.

- Make sure the temperature in the bedroom works for you. For me it needs to be quite cold in order to get the best sleep.

- Try to eat by 6.30pm to give your gut time to digest before bed. Or have at least a 2-hour window between eating and going to sleep.

- Ditch the caffeine and alcohol in the late evening.

Applying psychological techniques to stay positive

Physical activity, what you eat and how much sleep you get all play a huge role in combating anxiety and stress. Take the link between core body strength and stress control. Scientists now believe that activating core muscles such as your abdominal or back muscles helps to control the stress response system. To discover this, they had to inject monkeys with the rabies virus, which is unfortunate although that shouldn't detract from the findings. And it sheds new light on Pilates and yoga whose calming effects have long been thought to be psychological but may actually be physiological.

Stress for me means that my habits and systems are disordered. It could be a family row or a major work problem that sends you into turmoil and brings on those familiar feelings of anxiety. Everything you've embedded and have used to support yourself falls apart, from your morning weighing habit to logging your food intake. All those unconscious bad habits resurface, which in my case means picking food out of the fridge again or bingeing on half a loaf of bread.

The panicky feelings associated with anxiety can often be followed by a mental slump where you don't want to get out of bed in the morning. As I've said, winter 2021 was a particular low point for me. The dark nights and freezing days seemed to go on forever and the country was in lockdown just to make things appear even bleaker. And I'd put on weight after keeping it under control for so long. I wouldn't describe myself as a glass-half-empty person but this was the closest, I think, I've ever been to depression.

A staggering 264 million people globally are affected by depression, according to the World Health Organization. Depression is characterised by feeling sad persistently (not for a day but for days or weeks at a time) and displaying a lack of interest in activities or experiences you'd usually enjoy.

When you get low like this or stressed (which is often unavoidable), this can affect sleep and lead to dysfunctional eating habits. And when you're in that place, getting your routine back is an uphill struggle. Earlier in this book I said I treated sugar like an addict, and like someone who has been reliant on a drug, you will always be 'recovering'. The threat of sliding backwards never goes away, especially when you're stuck in a hastily-assembled home office faced with a new threat of being right by the fridge.

I found simple breathing techniques helpful during difficult times – and generally when I'm feeling overwhelmed. When I have a coffee in the morning, I will sit in a chair for a few minutes and practise them. They're also useful in a supermarket when I feel tempted 'just to have a browse' of the biscuit aisle.

By focusing on your breathing and getting it under control, you will find that the loud, critical voice in your head is gradually replaced by a quieter, more rational one. Then you can order your thoughts, be in the present moment and work out how you are going to complete the tasks ahead. The following are some straightforward methods to regain a sense of calm:

- **Four-square technique** – This powerful stress-buster is also known as 'box breathing'. Close your eyes, breathe in through your nose while counting to four slowly and feel the air fill your lungs. Next, hold your breath while again counting slowly to four. Exhale for four seconds. Repeat the steps ideally for four minutes in total.

- **Autogenic training** – A form of self-hypnosis, this approach gets you to focus attention on different areas of your body while practising simple phrases, such as 'My arms are warm' and 'My breathing is calm and regular'. This mind/body awareness allows you to switch off your 'fight, flight, freeze' responses.

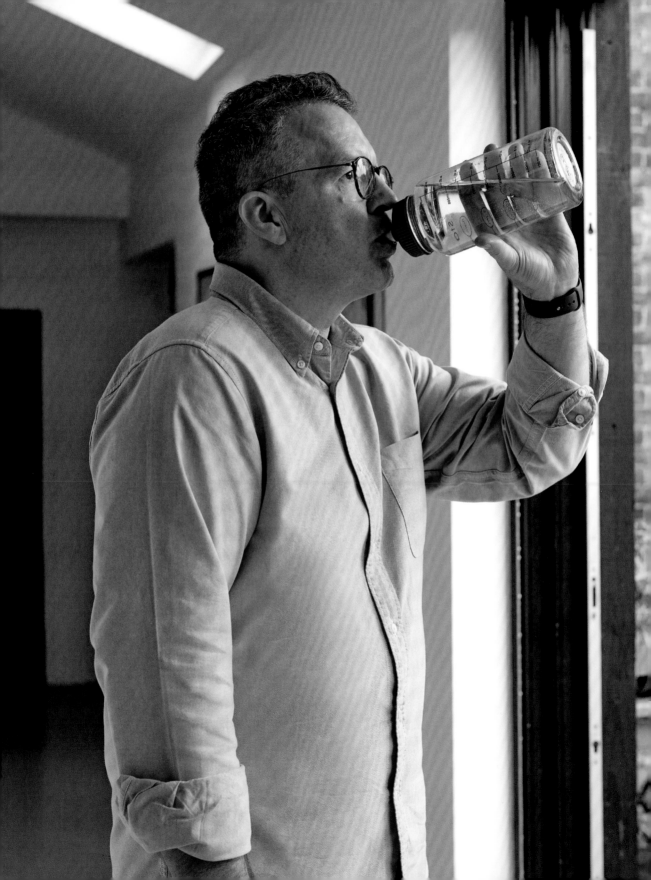

IN SUMMARY

- Don't panic when your clothes start to feel tight again – reset your routine if you're falling back into old ways.

- Moving house, changing job, caring for a relative are among the challenges that can throw you off course, so have an honest chat with yourself about what has unbalanced you.

- Get yourself a support network such as a walking group or exercise buddies to get you back on track.

- Surviving on fewer than 7 hours of sleep not only affects you mentally, it also impacts your weight, so set yourself a regular bedtime and stick to it.

- Ensure you truly believe your body and wellbeing are worth looking after.

- Try simple breathing exercises such as the Four-square technique to maintain a sense of calm and stop yourself spiralling downwards mentally.

- Never eat directly from the fridge or tell yourself you're just 'checking out the contents'.

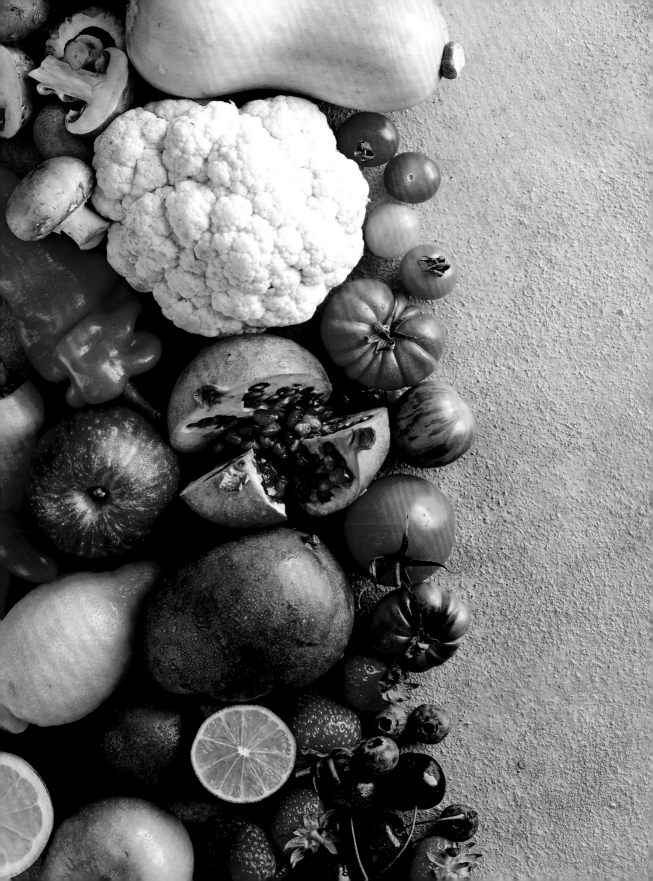

6 Recipes

When I look back on the food I used to eat, it's incomparable to what I consume today. Everything I eat now is tastier, more nutritious and more enjoyable to eat than the cheap pizzas, crappy microwave meals and ultra-processed gunge I used to throw into myself. The hardest thing to achieve when you dump ultra-processed food for real food is finding the time to prepare it. You have to be more organised with food shopping and meal planning, but the results are worth it. Over time, I built up a repertoire of standby meals. These recipes are easy and quick to make when you are pressed for time or short on ingredients. None of them is challenging to make. If they were, I wouldn't be cooking them. All of them are tasty. I hope you find these easy-to-cook recipes useful for your downsizing plan.

Carb swaps

Celeriac chips

Enjoy these low-carb vegetable chips instead of the usual potato variety and try them dipped in the Homemade mayonnaise (see page 167).

Serves 2

1 whole celeriac
2 tablespoons olive oil
1 teaspoon sea salt and/or 1 teaspoon Cajun seasoning

Preheat the oven to 200°C/gas mark 6 and pop a shallow baking tray in to preheat.

Remove the knobbly bits from the celeriac, peel, then slice it into rounds and then into chunky chips.

Toss the celeriac chips in a bowl with the olive oil and salt and/or Cajun seasoning and mix well.

Throw the oily seasoned chips into the preheated tray and bake for 25–30 minutes or until golden.

Carbohydrates – found in foods such as bread, rice, pasta, potatoes and yams – are calorie-dense because they are your body's primary fuel source. The body turns carbs into glucose for immediate energy, and stores excess as glycogen, and eventually fat, around the body. When you restrict the amount of carbs you eat over a sustained period, your body uses up its immediate energy stores, forcing it to burn fat reserves instead. This is why cutting out carbohydrates or severely reducing your intake is also advised for managing type 2 diabetes, as it helps to lower glucose levels in the blood and avoid spikes in blood sugar after meals.

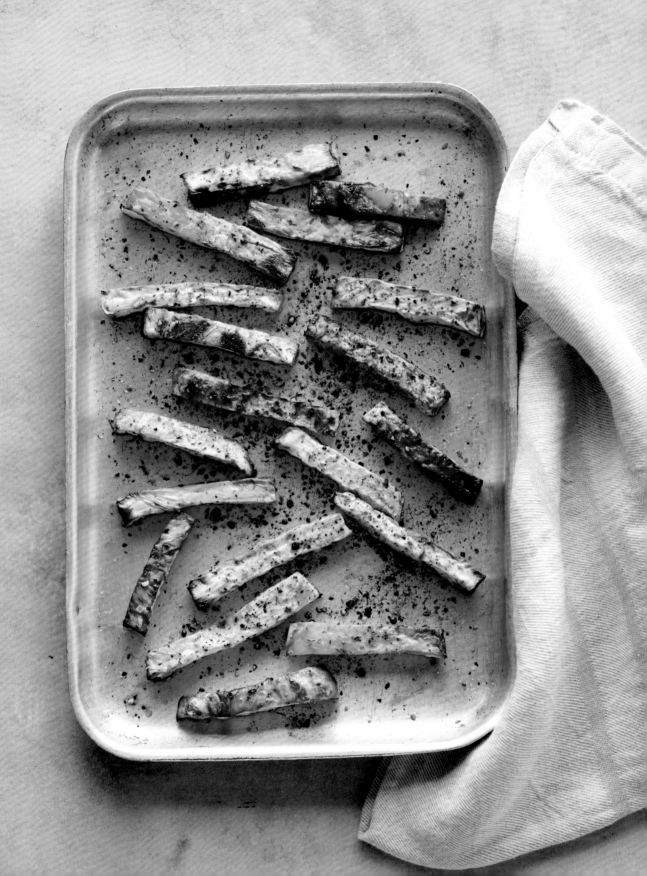

Cauliflower is a great
source of vitamin C, folate,
fibre and vitamin K.

Cauliflower/broccoli rice

All carbohydrates (starch, sugar and fibre) affect blood sugar levels but not all carbs are equal. Minimally processed wholegrains, such as brown rice, release energy more slowly than their more refined counterparts – white rice, pasta, bread – keeping you feeling full for longer. However, the best alternative for weight loss is cauliflower or broccoli rice, as both have far fewer calories than brown rice, with the added benefit of packing a greater nutritional punch. Studies have shown that eating more broccoli may lower the risk of heart disease by reducing the total amount of cholesterol in the body.

Serves 4

1 head of cauliflower or broccoli
1 teaspoon butter and/or olive oil
1 teaspoon water
salt and pepper

Cut the florets off the cauliflower or broccoli and blitz in a food processor until finely chopped.

Melt the butter and oil in a saucepan over a medium heat and add the cauliflower or broccoli rice, stirring well. Add the water and pop a lid on the pan, allowing the veg to steam. Cook for 5–10 minutes until tender.

Creamy cauliflower and broccoli cheese

This comfort food classic is also deliciously healthy with low-carb vegetables baked in a creamy, cheesy sauce.

Serves 4

1 head of cauliflower
1 head of broccoli
1 tablespoon butter
1 onion, finely chopped
1 teaspoon cumin seeds
1 teaspoon English mustard powder
200ml double cream
100g Cheddar cheese, grated
2 tablespoons almond flour
salt and pepper

Preheat the oven to 190°C/gas mark 5.

Steam the cauliflower and broccoli for about 10 minutes until slightly tender but firm.

Melt the butter in an ovenproof saucepan over a medium heat, add the onion and fry for 10 minutes until soft. Add the cumin seeds and mustard powder and cook for a few minutes before adding the cream and then three-quarters of the cheese. Add the veg to the cheesy cream. Combine the almond flour with the remaining cheese and sprinkle over the top.

Bake for 12–15 minutes until golden.

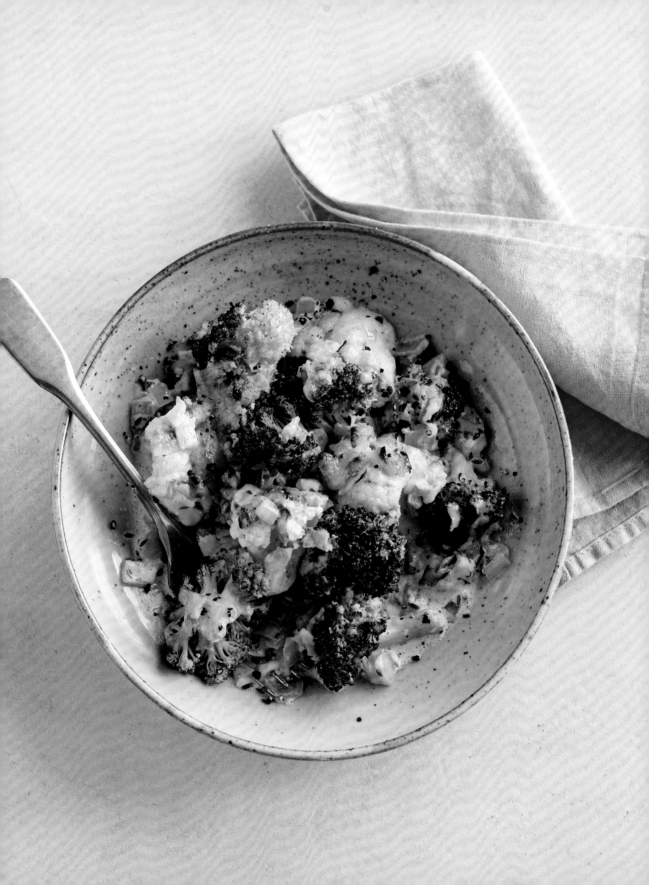

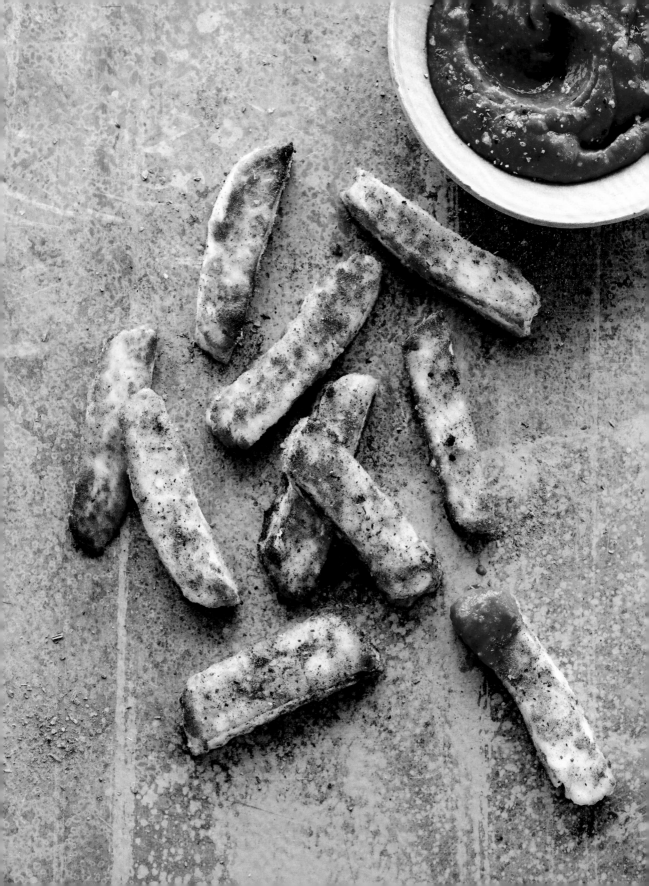

Halloumi chips

Great accompanied by the tomato sauce from the Weekend breakfast eggs (see page 154).

Serves 2

olive or avocado oil, for greasing
250g block halloumi cheese
1 egg
coconut or almond flour
garlic powder
Parmesan cheese, grated

Preheat the oven to 180°C/gas mark 4 and oil a baking tray.

Cut the halloumi into thick chips.

Beat the egg in a bowl and combine the dry ingredients in a separate bowl. Dip the halloumi chips into the beaten egg and then into the dry ingredients.

Place the halloumi chips on the oiled baking tray and bake for 20 minutes, or alternatively fry in a pan over high heat for 2 minutes, or until golden.

Courgetti

A great alternative to pasta, use courgetti with all your usual sauces, or add to salads like my Easy keto salad (see page 164).

Serves 2

4 courgettes
butter or olive oil, to taste
salt and pepper

Cut the courgettes to fit into your spiraliser and process to make long strands of courgetti.

Place the courgette strands in a colander or sieve set over a bowl and sprinkle with about 1 teaspoon of salt to extract some of the water – leave for 10 minutes.

Heat the butter or oil in a pan, add the courgetti and cook gently for 5 minutes. Season with salt and pepper to taste.

Courgettes are very low in calories but contain plenty of gut-friendly fibre (particularly in the skin), making them an ideal swap for starchy carbohydrates such as spaghetti. The soluble fibre in courgettes slows down digestion, helping to stabilise blood sugar and insulin levels, while the high water content helps the body to feel fuller faster. Courgettes also contain immune-system-boosting vitamin C, as well as potassium – which helps to control blood pressure.

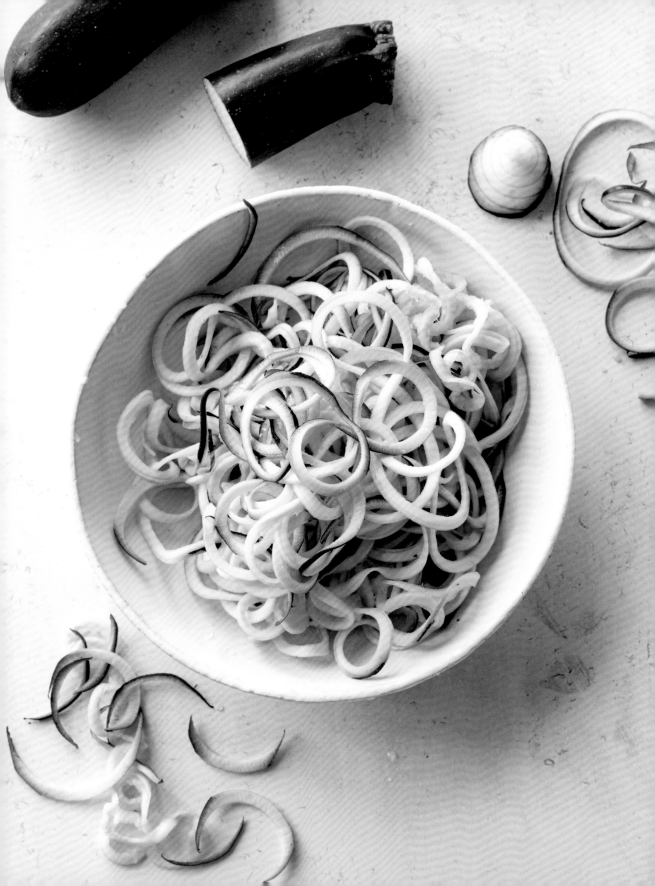

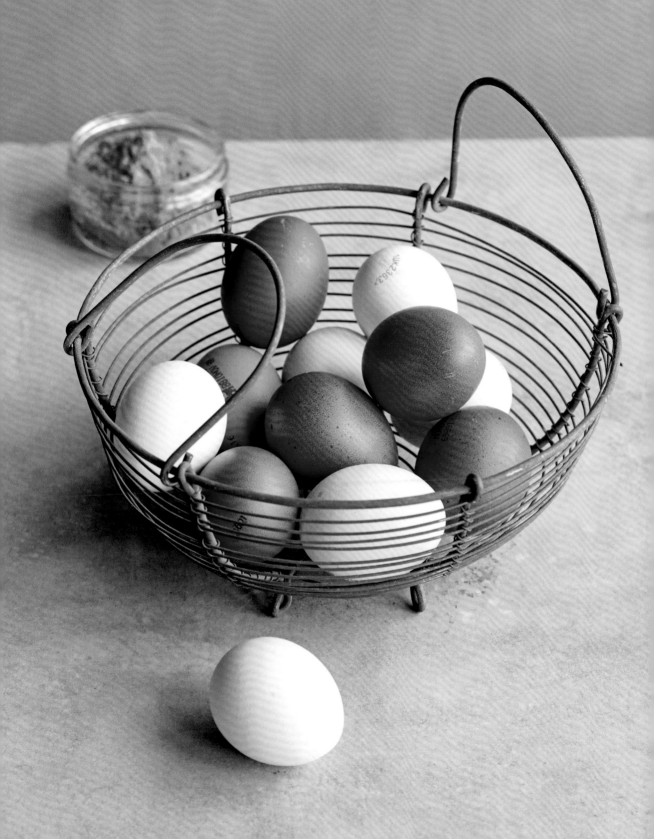

Easy eggs

Eggs are some of the most nutritionally complete foods out there; not only are they excellent sources of protein, on average containing 7g per egg, they are also naturally rich in vitamin B2, vitamin B12, vitamin D, vitamin A, iron, folate, selenium and iodine, as well as a whole host of other essential minerals needed by the body. Not a bad way to start the day!

Scrambled eggs with turmeric

Simple scrambled eggs with a hint of spice from the turmeric – great for breakfast, lunch or even a light dinner.

Serves 1

3 eggs
30ml double cream
1 teaspoon ground turmeric
1 tablespoon butter, plus extra to serve (optional)
salt and pepper

Beat the eggs and add the cream. Stir in the turmeric and season with salt and pepper.

Melt the butter in a heavy frying pan and stir in the egg mixture. Continue to stir until scrambled to your liking. Add a little more butter for extra butteriness.

Turmeric is natural source of curcumin – a powerful compound that gives the spice its distinguishable yellow hue as well as antioxidant and anti-inflammatory properties. Studies suggest that this compound can aid weight loss by suppressing fat tissue growth, as well as regulating blood sugar levels.

Just an omelette

Omelettes are so versatile – try this veggie version or experiment with your favourite fillings and try adding cooked meat or fish into the mix too.

Serves 1

3 eggs
butter
a large handful of spinach
6 medium-sized mushrooms, sliced
50g cheese of your choice, grated or sliced
salt and pepper

Preheat the oven to 190°C/gas mark 5.

Beat the eggs until frothy. Melt the butter in a heavy ovenproof frying pan set over a medium heat. Add the eggs and cook for 5–7 minutes until they have started to turn opaque, then add the spinach, mushrooms and then the cheese. Season and transfer the pan to the oven for 2–10 minutes until the omelette is set and golden.

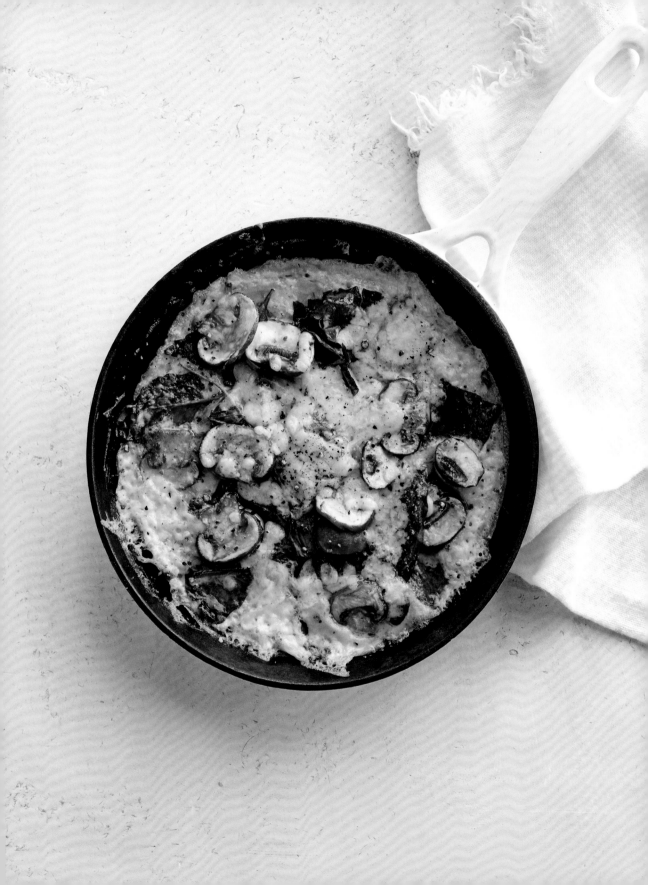

Weekend breakfast eggs

This takes a bit of time to prepare, but it is well worth the wait. I make it most weekends as a special treat. The tomatoes are great served with the Halloumi chips on page 147.

Serves 4 or 2 hungry diners

2 punnets of cherry tomatoes
1 red onion, cut into wedges
1 red pepper
3 garlic cloves
a pinch of chilli flakes
a squeeze of lemon juice
4 eggs
100g feta cheese
fresh coriander, chopped
salt and pepper

Preheat the oven to 190°C/gas mark 5.

Dry-fry the whole tomatoes, onion wedges, unpeeled garlic and whole pepper in an ovenproof frying pan on a high heat for 3–4 minutes until blackened on the edges. Remove from the heat and leave to cool slightly.

Squeeze out the flesh from the unpeeled garlic into a processor and whizz up with the tomatoes and onion until relatively smooth. Return the mixture to the frying pan and simmer for 10 minutes on a low heat to reduce it a little. Dice the pepper into 2cm pieces, removing the seeds, and add to the mixture to soften a little more. Add the chilli flakes and season with a bit of salt and pepper.

Add a squeeze of lemon juice and make four wells in the mixture with the back of a spoon. Break an egg into each one. Pop the pan in the oven for 10 minutes until the eggs are no longer runny. Crumble over the feta and coriander and serve.

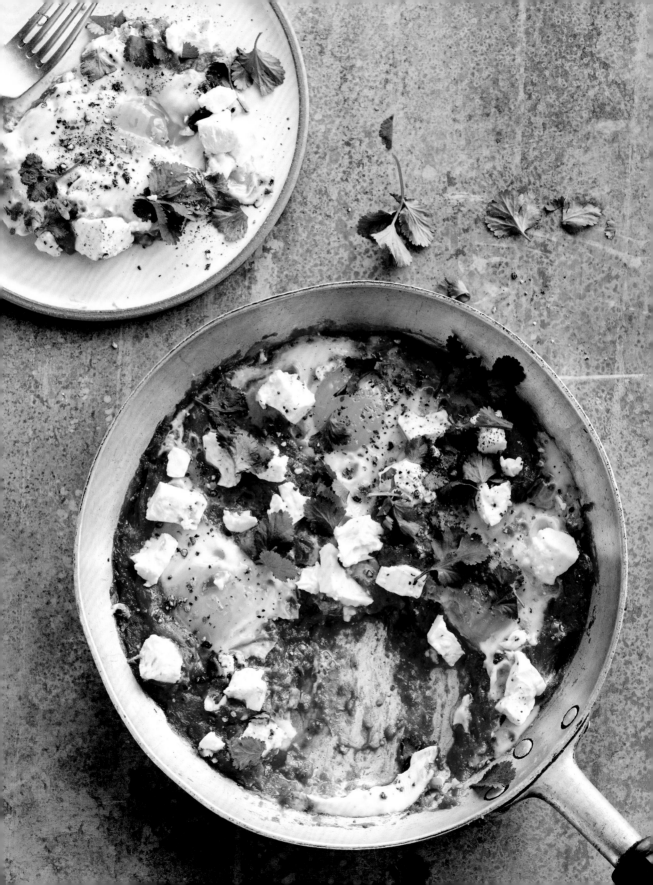

Egg and bacon muffins

A new way to enjoy your morning bacon and eggs.

Serves 2–3

1 tablespoon coconut oil, melted
6 slices of bacon or ham
6 eggs
75g cheese, grated
salt and pepper

Preheat the oven to 200°C/gas mark 6.

Oil a 6-hole muffin tin with the oil or line with baking paper. Line each hole with a slice of bacon or ham. Crack an egg into each one, season with salt and pepper and sprinkle over the cheese. Bake for about 15 minutes.

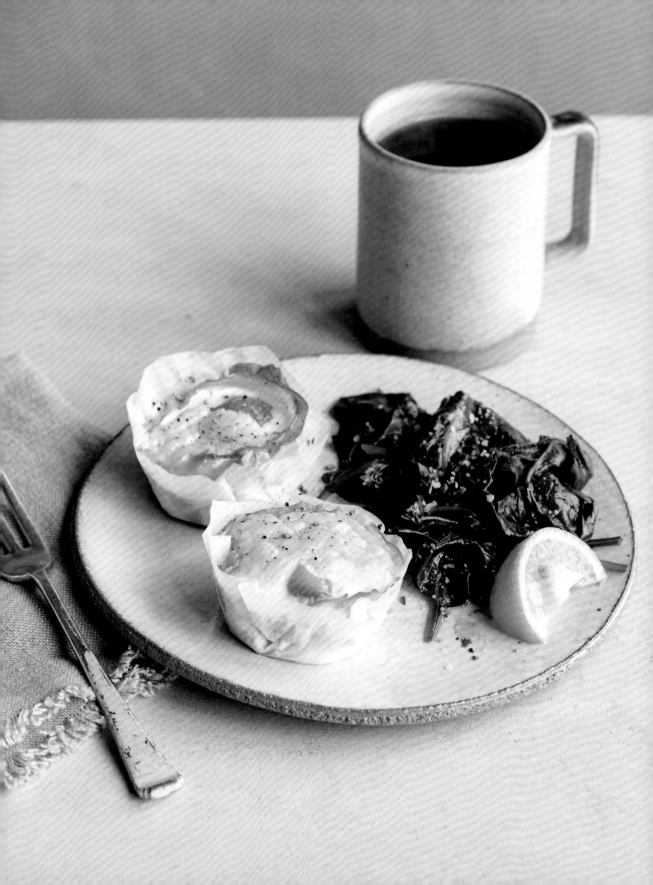

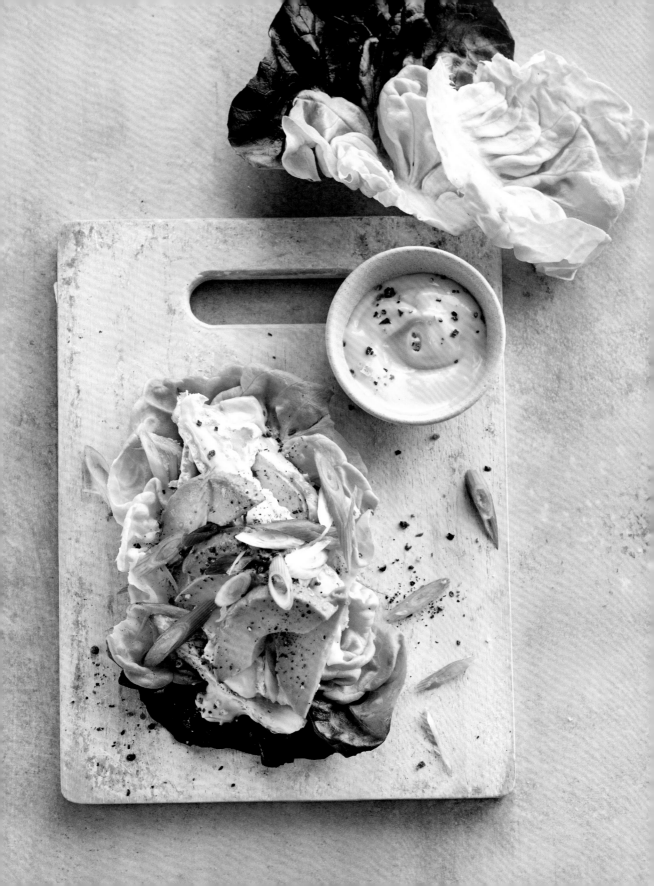

Easy fixes

Can't-wait-any-longer sandwich

When I get hunger cravings and just need to eat, using the leaves of a big lettuce instead of bread is my go-to meal. It works in Five Guys burgers too.

Serves 1

4 big lettuce leaves
2 teaspoons Homemade mayonnaise (see page 167) or mayo made with avocado oil (available online and in good supermarkets)
2 spring onions, sliced
90g cooked chicken or turkey
½ avocado, thinly sliced
30g Brie, sliced
salt and pepper

Spread out the lettuce leaves, overlapping each other. Using a lettuce with soft leaves rather than the crispy type is best. Spread two of the lettuce leaves with half the mayo and scatter over the sliced spring onions. Top with the meat, sliced avocado and Brie. Add salt and pepper and the remaining mayo.

Top with the two remaining lettuce leaves. It's a little messy, so you'll need a plate, but it tastes great. You're eating quickly prepared nutritious food, and you've avoided bread.

Whole roasted Romanesco cauliflower

When I started eating keto and low-carb meals, I was always deficient in easy-to-prepare but tasty vegetable recipes. If you are going low-carb or keto, at some point you'll have to learn to enjoy cauliflower and broccoli. I honestly love both vegetables these days, but they do take a bit of getting used to.

Serves 2–3 per cauliflower

1 or 2 whole Romanesco cauliflowers
olive oil, for drizzling
50g Parmesan cheese, grated
1 teaspoon smoked paprika
1 lemon, quartered
salt and pepper

Preheat the oven to 200°C/gas mark 6.

Steam the cauliflower(s) for 10 minutes until just about tender. Place in a roasting tin and drizzle with olive oil. Sprinkle over the Parmesan and paprika and season with a bit of salt and pepper. Place the lemon wedges alongside the cauli(s).

Roast for 25 minutes until golden. When cooked a little, squeeze over the roasted lemon juice. Cut the cauliflower(s) into wedges to serve.

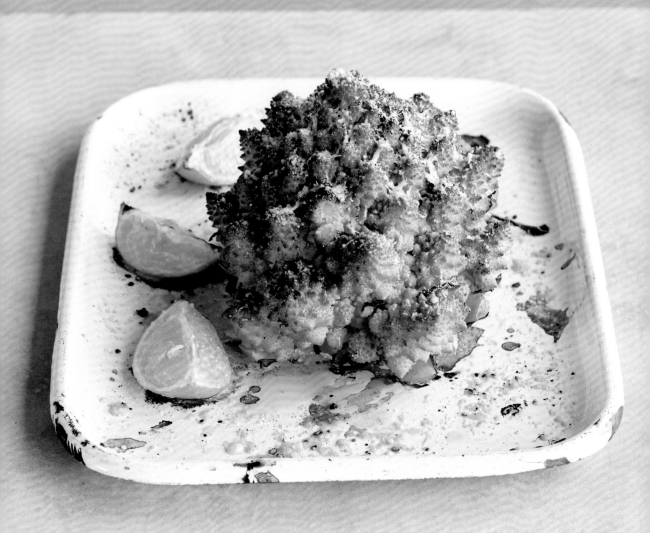

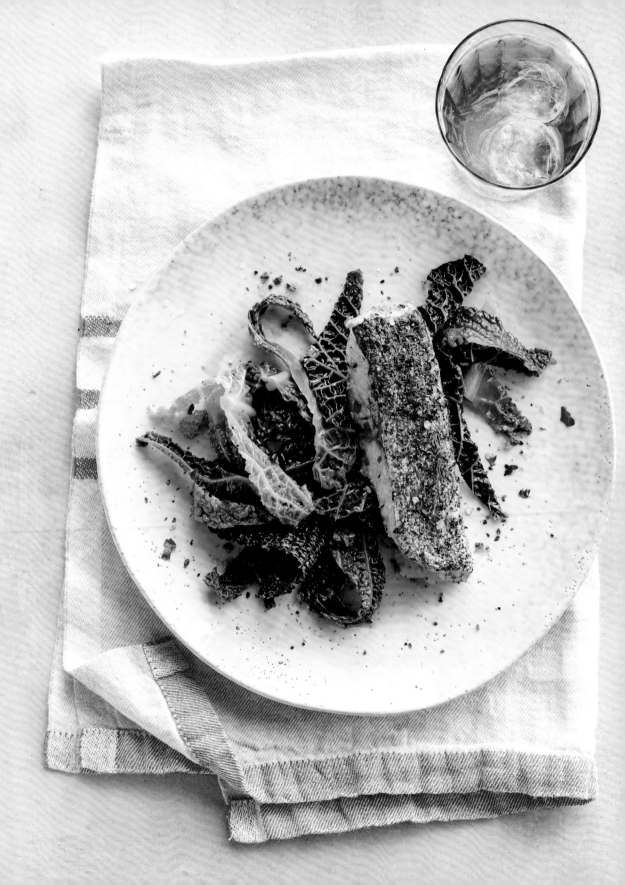

Spiced salmon

This is a really simple and quick-to-prepare keto dinner. There are endless variations of things you can do with salmon, but this is my favourite.

Serves 2

olive oil, for greasing
½ teaspoon allspice
1 teaspoon garlic powder
½ teaspoon ground cinnamon
½ teaspoon black pepper
1 teaspoon cayenne pepper
1½ teaspoons dried thyme
a pinch of chilli flakes
½ teaspoon sukrin gold (optional)
4 salmon fillets, skin on

Preheat the oven to 200°C/gas mark 6 and oil a baking tray.

Mix all the dry ingredients together and coat the salmon on all sides. Place the salmon on the oiled baking tray, skin-side up, and cook for 20 minutes or until the salmon is cooked through and the skin is a little crispy.

Serve with shredded cabbage sautéed in butter with a tablespoon of water added and steamed for a few minutes. Season well with salt and black pepper.

Easy keto salad

I throw this together at least once a week. It's low-carb, low-calorie, quick to make and tastes great.

Serves 2

145g tin of tuna in brine or spring water, drained
1 tablespoons Homemade mayonnaise (see page 167) or mayo made with avocado oil (available online and in good supermarkets)
3 spring onions, thinly sliced
2 portions of Courgetti (see page 148)
olive oil, for drizzling
3 tomatoes, sliced
3 hard-boiled eggs, quartered
salt and pepper

Mix the tuna, mayo and spring onions together and season with salt and pepper. Toss your thinly spiralised courgetti in a bowl with olive oil and another sprinkle of salt and pepper. Divide between two bowls and top with the tomatoes, eggs and tuna.

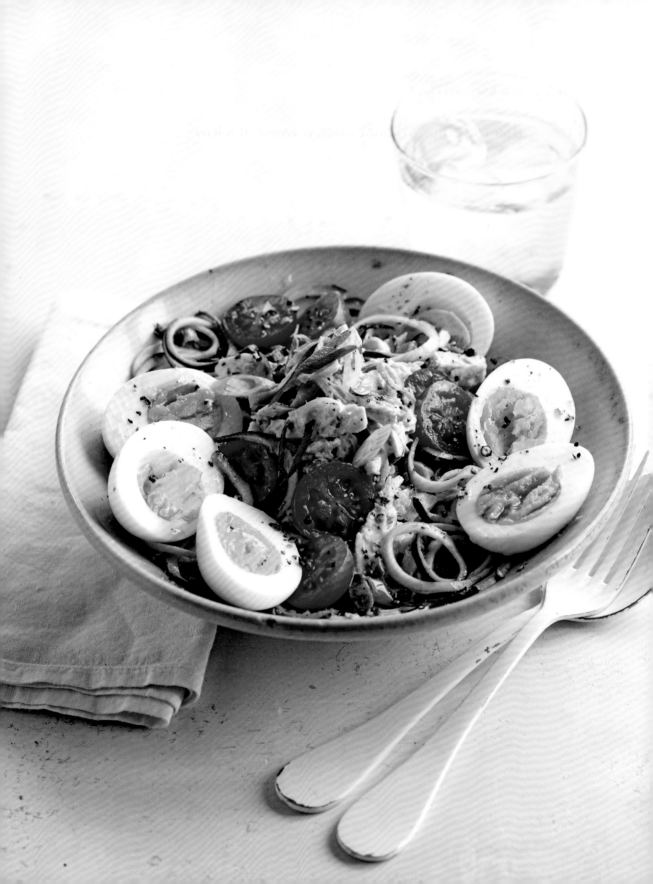

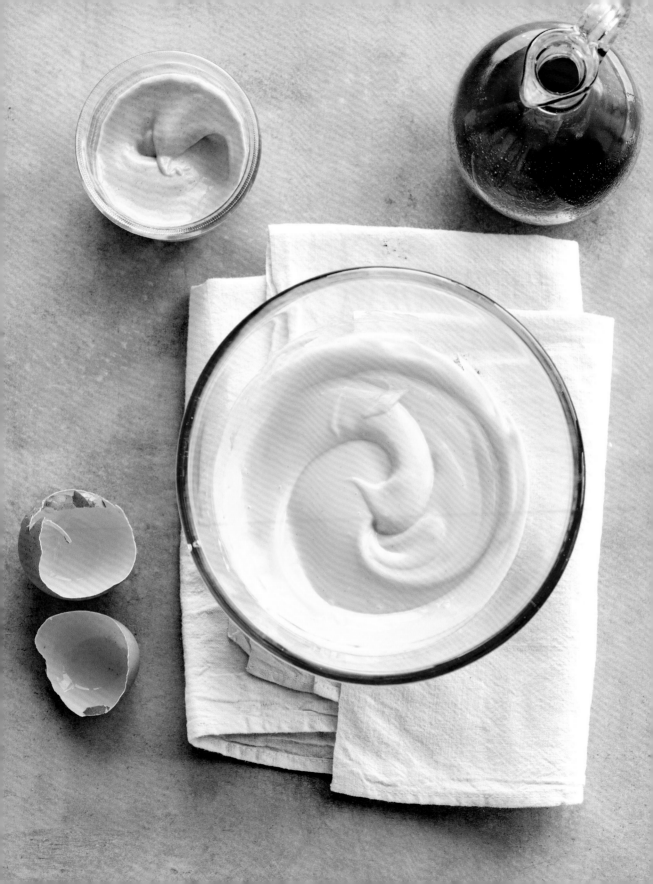

Homemade mayonnaise

Making your own mayo is simple, but it's a bit of a faff. It's worth it though as it goes with nearly everything in your new repertoire of food. If I'm not in the mood to make it, I always have a jar of Hunter & Gather mayonnaise made with avocado oil in the fridge. It's a bit pricier than typical mayo, but it's richer, and you need less of it. If you're in the mood, though, make your own and experiment with different flavours – I often add a tablespoon of curry powder to spice it up.

1 large egg
1 teaspoon Dijon mustard
2 teaspoons white wine vinegar
250ml olive or avocado oil

Crack the egg into a high bowl or measuring jug and add the mustard and vinegar. Using a stick blender with the whirring bit at the bottom of the bowl, slowly pour in the oil in a steady stream. It takes a bit of practice to get this right but start with the blender at the bottom and slowly lift it up. You should be OK without it splattering everywhere. When it's blended, add more vinegar or mustard, depending on taste. The mixture will last about 5 days if you keep it in the fridge – I store it in an old jam jar with a screw-top lid.

Resources

Many gurus and guides have assisted me in my journey to get healthy – a huge thank you to them all. A selection of those either referenced in the book or that added to my thinking are listed below:

Michael Mosley *The Fast Diet* and *The 8-Week Blood Sugar Diet*

David Goggins *Can't Hurt Me*

David Moss *Salt, Sugar, Fat: How the Food Giants Hooked Us*

Aseem Malhotra and Donal O'Neill *The Pioppi Diet: A 21-Day Plan to Lose Weight and Live Longer, Happier and Healthier*

Dave Asprey *The Bulletproof Diet: Lose Up to a Pound a Day, Reclaim Your Energy and Focus, and Upgrade Your Life*

Professor Luigi Fontana *The Path to Longevity: How to Reach 100 with the Health and Stamina of a 40-Year-Old*

Professor Edith Hall *Aristotle's Way: How Ancient Wisdom Can Change Your Life*

B.J. Fogg *Tiny Habits: The Small Changes That Change Everything*

Vybarr Cregan-Reid *Primate Change: How the world we made is remaking us*

James Clear *Atomic Habits: An Easy and Proven Way to Build Good Habits and Break Bad Ones*

Professor Matthew Walker *Why We Sleep*

Caroline Williams *Move!:The New Science of Body Over Mind*

Shane O'Mara *In Praise of Walking: The New Science of How We Walk and Why It's Good for Us*

Professor Matthew Walker *Why We Sleep: The New Science of Dreams*

Dr Jen Unwin *Fork in the Road: A Hopeful Guide to Food Freedom*

Olli Sovijarvi *The Biohackers Handbook: Upgrade Yourself and Unleash Your Inner Potential*

Dr Valter Longo *The Longevity Diet*

Gareth Leng *The Heart of the Brain: The Hypothalamus and Its Hormones*

Dave Asprey *Bulletproof: The Cookbook*

Niaamh Shields *Bacon: The Cookbook*

Mark Sissons *The Keto Reset Diet*

Dr Josh Axe *Keto Diet Cookbook*

Colonel Arthur R Kenney-Herbert Fifty *Breakfasts: A Splendid Victorian Collection of over 130 Classic Breakfast Recipes*

John Meechan and Ally Houston *Paleo Canteen Low Carb on a Budget*

Kate Caldesi *The Diabetes Weightloss Cookbook: A life-changing diet to prevent and reverse type 2 diabetes*

Monya Kilian Palmer *Keto Kitchen: Delicious recipes for energy and weight loss*

Resources and recipes for low-carb and keto lifestyles: www.dietdoctor.com

Index

Acknowledgements

I find writing books more stressful than politics, which is why I am incredibly grateful to my editor, Judith Hannam, for her kindness and patience. Judith encouraged me to produce *Lose Weight 4 Life* after the success of my previous book *Downsizing*, co-written with Jo Lake. Jo and I were taken aback by the many readers' questions about how I reorganised my life to lose weight and regain my health.

Without Judith and the team at Kyle books, including Joanna Copestick, Caroline Brown, Megan Brown and Samhita Foria, I would never have started this project. I'm grateful, too, to the photographer Peter Cassidy and the designer, Paul Palmer-Edwards.

Thank you also to the sagacious Rory Scarfe and the team at The Neil Blair Partnership for their support and representation.

My team, Lucy Pullin, Jeff Courtney, Jo Watson and Sophie Goodchild, have been helpful and supportive through multiple lockdowns, family health scares and bereavements. This book would never have made it to the printers without them, particularly Sophie. I am immensely grateful.

When my steps target began to drop during the Covid lockdowns, my partner Sarah Perrett decided that this was because we lacked a dog in our lives. I now have a four-legged personal trainer called Fugee. Thank you, Sarah. There is plenty of research that suggests owning a dog increases longevity. Let's hope so! Sarah's kids, Gabriel, Rafa, Manny and my kids, Malachy and Saoirse, have, in their unique ways, encouraged me to keep going when lockdown cheese-eating nearly got the better of me. Thank you and much love to each of them.

In my last book, I credited the changes I made to various clinicians, scientists, writers, and biohackers who have profoundly impacted my life. I remain grateful to my GP, Dr Shaukat Nazeer, Clare Nasir, Max Wind Cowie, Dr Michael Mosley, Professor David Sinclair, Dr Matthew Walker, Dr Aseem Malhotra, Dr Jeff Volek, Dr Stephen Phinney, Dr Jennifer Unwin, Dr David Unwin, Dave Asprey and Peter Attia MD.

I couldn't have made the changes to my lifestyle without the support of Baroness Alicia Kennedy. She gave me the inspiration to carry on. Since publishing my last book, Alicia has been on her own health journey. I'm proud of her.

Final thanks go to the hundreds of people who have written and emailed or stopped me in the street to give encouragement and feedback, especially my many friends and neighbours in Bewdley and Kidderminster.

Also by Tom Watson

Downsizing: How I lost 8 stone, reversed my diabetes and regained my health

'On 8 January 2017, I celebrated my 50th birthday, marking the milestone by throwing a knees-up for friends at the Rivoli Ballroom in South-East London. The following morning, I woke up nursing the mother of all hangovers. Fifty and fab! Proclaimed one of my birthday cards. Fifty and fat!, more like I thought.'

Tom Watson began to put on weight in his early twenties, having developed an appetite for fast food and cheap beer while studying at the University of Hull. As time progressed – and his penchant for anything sweet, fatty or fizzy persisted – he found himself adjusting his belt, loosening his collar and upsizing his wardrobe to XXL. He continued to pile on the pounds when he entered the world of politics as MP for West Bromwich East (despite short-lived flirtations with fad diets and fitness classes). By December 2014, his bathroom scales had tipped to 22 stone. After being diagnosed with type 2 diabetes in late 2015, he decided to take control of his diet and exercise. He started to feel better quickly and within a short time his long-term blood sugar levels were within normal range. By July 2018, he came off medication.

Praise for *Downsizing*:

'An honest and fascinating account of the journey that Tom made from discovering he was a type 2 diabetic to doing something about it. This book will change lives.'
Michael Mosley

'Enjoyable for stories of Watson's high stress/high booze/poor sleep/comfort eating political life'
The Times

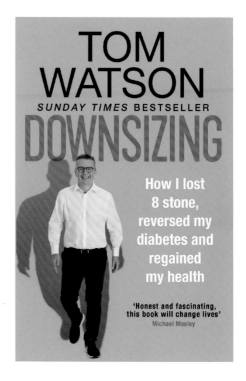